Guiding Our Parents in the Right Direction

Practical Advice about Seniors Moving From the Home They Love

BRUCE NEMOVITZ

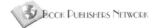

BOOK PUBLISHERS NETWORK

Book Publishers Network
P.O. Box 2256
Bothell • WA • 98041
PH • 425-483-3040
www.bookpublishersnetwork.com

10 9 8 7 6 5 4 3 2 1

Printed in the United States of America

LCCN   2013944969
ISBN   978-1-937454-93-7

Editor: Julie Scandora
Cover design: Laura Zugzda
Interior design: Stephanie Martindale
Photo: Generations Family Unpacking Boxes Moving House © Darren Baker | Dreamstime.com

To my mother who showed me the way

To my wife who showed me the stars

To my children who showed me the wonder

To my grandchildren who showed me the why

I can fight, rebel, and even resent what is happening, or I can surrender to "what is" and focus all of my energy on creating something better.

Og Mandino
Today I Begin a New Life

Contents

HOW THIS BOOK WILL HELP YOU   ix

ACKNOWLEDGMENTS   xi

INTRODUCTION   xiii
The Murray Family's Story

CHAPTER ONE:
ROLE FOR CHILDREN OF SENIORS   1
Communicating with Family
Understanding Your Parents
Getting Both Parents to Communicate
The Murray Family's Story

CHAPTER TWO:
IT'S ALL IN THE MIND   11
Changing the Story
Keeping an Open Attitude
Confronting the Options
The Murray Family's Story

CHAPTER THREE:
  WHY MOVE?   25
  Getting Your Parents Receptive to Considering a Move
  Listing Pros and Cons
  Taking Emotional Inventory
  The Murray Family Story

CHAPTER FOUR:
  SOLVING THE UNSPOKEN PROBLEM   33
  Remaining Independent
  Facing Downsizing
  Dealing with Uncertainty
  Facing Our Feelings
  Tom's Story

CHAPTER FIVE:
  CHOOSING WISELY   47
  Seeking Friendly Advice
  Asking the Experts
  Looking at Housing Options
  The Murray Family's Story

CHAPTER SIX:
  CREATING THE HOUSING PLAN   63
  What Do Your Parents Really Want?
  A Housing Plan
  Details of the Housing Plan
  Summary

CHAPTER SEVEN:
  DOWNSIZING   73
  Letting Go Emotionally
  Sorting
  Distributing Possessions
  Using Professionals
  Handling the Physical Job
  The Murray Family's Story

CHAPTER EIGHT:
SELECTING A REALTOR 87
Advantages of a Senior Real Estate Specialist
Interviewing Realtors

CHAPTER NINE:
PRICING THE HOME 91
Consider the Source
The Competition
As-is Cash Sale
Selling As-is versus Making Improvements

CHAPTER TEN:
PREPARING THE HOME FOR SALE 103
Reasons to Improve the Home
Prioritizing Work on the House
Staging a Home
What to Do Now
The Murray Family's Story

CHAPTER ELEVEN:
SELLING THE HOME 115
Timing the Sale
Presenting the Home
Home Inspection
Moving Out
The Murray Family's Story
Shirley's Story

ABOUT THE AUTHOR 131

HOW THIS BOOK
WILL HELP YOU

THIS BOOK IS designed to be used as a "toolbox" to assist you in helping your parents' transition from their long-time home to the next step in their lives. Each "tool," or chapter, is intended to give you the information you will need to successfully guide your loved ones to their new home and help avoid common mistakes and pitfalls in the process.

Though you may choose to read the book from the beginning, it is designed as a resource guide for you to consult as each situation calls for the information and insights needed at that time.

To help your parents, while you read this book, you may want to let them read my previous book, *Moving in the Right Direction, A Senior's Guide to Moving and Downsizing.* It addresses many points I bring up in this one but from their point of view. Letting them read that guide on their own may prepare them for what you must discuss with them. Just leaving *Moving in the Right Direction* with your parents allows them to think about difficult subjects on their terms—at the time they want, at the pace they prefer, with no one forcing issues upon them.

Whether you use *Guiding Our Parents in the Right Direction* alone or with *Moving in the Right Direction*, you will have important advice for guiding your parents. Most important, you will gain a perspective from your parents' points of view, which will support your efforts to become a better listener and advocate throughout the process so that everyone comes out ahead.

ACKNOWLEDGMENTS

MY THANKS TO Adele Lund for persevering with me as my advisor throughout the entire process of gathering information and organizing this book.

I am especially grateful to the families who have contributed their stories with their memories and experiences. My thanks go also to the many senior communities who have given me a platform to gather information from children of seniors who were in the process of moving their loved ones to their new homes.

I thank my friend Ed, who always provides the insights needed to understand others.

My gratitude goes to my mother, Millie, my children, Dara and Karra, and my grandchildren, who constantly remind me about the importance of family and love for one another. To my sister, Sharon, and brothers, Paul and Howard, and their families for their constant support. Most of all, I thank my wife, Jeanne, who helps me to understand the value of each day and the uniqueness of each individual. Her optimism and hope to help families kept me moving forward with this project.

INTRODUCTION

THE CALL COMES in, and a stressed voice on the other end is asking for a sympathetic ear, for direction, and for hope in a situation that many times may feel overwhelming with no apparent end in sight. The child of a senior needs help with a parent or parents. So many children are faced with parents who enjoyed living many years in the home where they raised their families and now must leave to move into housing that meets their current needs. The children want the best for their parents, but they do not know how to begin the process.

When I began my real estate practice thirty-five years ago, my learning curve had just begun. I would walk into so many different types of situations compelling people to buy or sell a home—the death of a spouse, divorce, first-time homebuyers, downsizing to a smaller home, and so many other reasons. Over time, I felt a call towards helping seniors with their unique set of circumstances that were not being addressed by anyone—not by me or any other Realtor in the industry. Older adults who had lived in their homes for many years were overwhelmed with the thought of moving from their long-time home and seemed paralyzed when trying to cope with this major change to finding suitable housing. I made the decision about twenty years ago to focus my real estate sales business on those seniors who needed more than a Realtor—an advisor who could offer the tools necessary to make a move that was necessary as their homes no longer met their physical and mental needs. I wrote my first book, *Moving in the Right Direction, A Senior's Guide to Moving and Downsizing* to give such advice. The book has been read by thousands, and I have received so many positive letters and emails from my readers thanking me for identifying with their fears, hopes, and desires to find new housing to meet their current needs.

Since the release of my first book, I realized a shift was occurring related to the calls I was receiving. More and more of the calls were coming from the children of seniors. These calls more times than not were distressed voices in need of immediate help. Their parents had waited too long in their homes. Age waits for no one and no thing, especially a market change! A parent would succumb to a fall or major health change, such as Alzheimer's, stroke, or other debilitating disease. The children were as overwhelmed as the parents I had met before publishing my first book. However, the children's challenges in helping their parents were somewhat different from the set of circumstances facing their parents. Taking care of their own families with children while helping their parents at the same time was truly daunting. Add to that the dynamics between siblings, each with different ideas of what to do with the senior parents, and you have a recipe for confusion, frustration, and not knowing which way to turn.

Therefore, my intent for this book is to provide the coping mechanisms, tools, and strategies for you to use in helping make a successful move for your parents. I have also addressed the topic of coping with family issues between siblings, as well as an understanding and perspective from your parents' point of view. My goal is that you will know what services are available to help assist in this transition, as well as providing answers to the many questions and concerns when helping assist those you love so dearly ... your parent or parents!

THE MURRAY FAMILY'S STORY

RECENTLY, I HAD the pleasure of working with a wonderful family as they transitioned their elder parents from their home of many years to a senior community. Because I was so moved by the way they navigated this process, I asked the three daughters if they would allow me to share their story with you. They graciously accepted. Although we have changed their names and other identifying information, all that happened is true and in their own words. You will find their story unfold throughout the book at the end of some of the chapters. Let me introduce you to them.

We are three daughters in a very typical and loving family of five. Both parents are nearly ninety. They grew up during the Great Depression and married after WWII when Dad returned home from the war. Throughout the years, they have been very independent. Both still are involved with their church. They value being active and independent as this is a very important part of keeping them mentally and physically fit. Until last year, they mall-walked, and Dad kept busy with yard work while Mom hung out the wash, navigating the basement stairs with wash basket in hand. Dad still hunts and fishes, and Mom still cooks, bakes, knits and quilts.

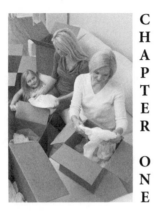

CHAPTER ONE

ROLE FOR CHILDREN OF SENIORS

ALTHOUGH THE SOURCE of many of my distress calls has shifted from seniors to children of seniors, the reasons for the calls remain the same. A health change has forced hasty decisions that have led to unhappiness and sadness.

Now, the children of seniors have to make the decision for parents that have stayed too long in an environment inappropriate for their needs. By delaying making a move, the parents are forced into a situation done with little planning due to the urgency of the moment. This has led to the family of the older adult burdened with the pressures of selling the home and determining where their loved one will spend the rest of their days.

No parent would ever wish this responsibility to be placed upon a child or family. However, by waiting too long, the family becomes one in crisis, and too often, siblings can turn on each other in the attempt to make the right decisions for their parents.

It is important to focus on creating a housing plan for your parents well before crisis hits. Despite good intentions, some of you may still find yourselves thrown into turmoil and having to get immediate housing for your parents. You will deal with the same issues ... but at hyper speed.

Whether you have the luxury of time in working with your parents on a plan for living arrangements or must react with lightning speed, the best approach to manage the myriad decisions involves organizing the steps you must take and tackling them one at a time. To make the process as smooth as possible, one of your first steps takes you to communicating with the rest of the family.

Communicating with Family

Communication is critical when faced with such a daunting situation as finding the proper fit of housing for your parents, as well as their downsizing after years of accumulation. And you must involve all important members of the family—your siblings, your parents, and trusted advisors. There are financial concerns and medical issues as well. In many cases, the parents may have some medical challenges and cannot contribute to the move as they would like. So that voice calling me for help feels alone and frustrated! Communication is essential, but where does the advice and guidance originate?

If you have siblings, you undoubtedly spent many years living with them and know them very well, maybe even too well, and may want to keep some of them out of the discussion about housing for Mom and Dad. Take care if you do so. Each family has its own dynamics, but open communication among all relevant members, although difficult to wade through, usually makes for a better outcome for all concerned.

Invariably, siblings will have differing views about how best to care for their aging parents. I have had the honor to work with many families who have struggled through the process of helping parents transition from single-family home living to a senior apartment or community. In the end, the majority of the siblings

I work with have one goal, and that is to make sure their parents are safe and secure with the best quality of life.

Still, with complicated connections between brothers and sisters, confusion and sometimes disagreements may occur when trying to help Mom and Dad.

In addition, the parents may have strong ideas about how much to involve their children. Many of my seniors choose not to involve their children. Others will not make any decisions without involving at least one child. Some want a consensus of all children before deciding what their best options are. You can see that one size does not fit all when senior parents need to consider a significant change, such as a move to new housing.

To add to the complex family dynamics, often one of the children has the burden of most or all decisions for the parents and is then subject to criticism from the other siblings. In other situations, siblings living in other cities or states tend to want solutions quickly, based on a holiday visit. Because they live far away and do not see Mom or Dad on a daily basis, when they do visit, the physical changes in their parents become much more pronounced. The result is a feeling of urgency to get their parents immediately out of an unhealthy situation, leaving much of the work to the siblings who live closest to Mom or Dad. This situation can lead to damaged relationships and lasting animosity between siblings.

At the same time, the children often have strong emotional attachments to their parents' home. Despite recognizing the parents' needs for a move, the children may cry, "It's just not fair." We children never want to see our childhood home sold to someone else, to some family that has no idea of the history of this bastion of emotion, to people who have no meaningful connection to the place.

This is the case for so many of us. We just assumed Mom and Dad would never sell the home that provided our safety and happiness for so many years. Well, like the inevitable change of seasons, the time has come for a major change in our parents' lives, as well as in our lives as their children. As with any change, how we get through it will depend on the way in which we choose to view this event.

This is the time to put Mom and Dad's self-interests first. In many cases, it is only Mom or only Dad now. Just think of how difficult this decision is for a single senior now without a spouse. It is hard enough for a couple that has stronger emotional connections to the home than do any of their children. This decision had been a labored one, involving many days of anguish and uncertainty. This is the time to put your feelings aside and think of the well-being and happiness of your parents. It has been my experience throughout my career that most children of seniors do put their parents' self-interest in front of their own. But in some cases, I have witnessed the opposite, where the children have reverted to banging their heads against the wall in protest, just as they did when they were young, living at home with their parents.

Take time to assess the true needs of your parents. Would a move be beneficial for them? Would they be closer to the rest of the family, providing a safer situation in case of emergency? Would this new location offer services and choices they currently lack? If you put yourself in their place, would you want to stay where they now are, or would you want to move to a new location? Does the family home currently meet all of their physical demands? Are you willing to help with the everyday maintenance of their home, or are you too busy with your own family and home to help? These are questions you need to ask before you let your emotions run away from the reality of the situation at hand.

After you answer these questions honestly, you may find that a move is not only needed but also an immediate necessity. Once you come to this realization, then the loss of your childhood home becomes the gain for Mom and Dad, as well as the only solution for the entire family. You will always have the memories of growing up, and most important, you will have your parents in a safe and healthy environment.

Understanding Your Parents

It is especially critical to understand the parents' feelings, fears, anxieties, and wishes for their future. All too often, the children of older adults make assumptions based on their lives and their experiences when making statements and suggestions to siblings and their parents. Parents become frustrated with their children when solutions and goals are determined without the input of the person actually moving.

Many of my senior clients tell me that their children mean well and want the best for their safety and well-being but do not understand how they feel about moving to a new environment. They do not and cannot understand how overwhelming thoughts of moving, downsizing, and living in an unknown environment can be. It is especially challenging when they have been in their homes for so many years living independently from their children.

Try to better understand their viewpoint and feelings. This is what I often hear:

"My kids don't understand!"

"It's my safety zone."

"I've lived here for forty years."

"This home is my memories, not just a building and foundation."

"It's hard to think of moving to a community and having to make new friends." "What if my money runs out? Will they kick me out?"

"How do I start going through everything? … There's so much."

"I don't want to burden my family … but I don't have anyone to help me."

"What if I move and I hate it?"

Over the course of my career in working with seniors and their families, the above questions and comments have been a constant when dealing with moves of seniors from their long-time home. Some have described the stress of moving as somewhere between a divorce and a colonoscopy. Ouch! As we age, change becomes more and more difficult. As children of seniors, we want the best for our parents. We want them in a safe and thriving environment so that peace of mind can be achieved for both children and their parents.

Communication is so important in a successful move, and all too often, our best intentions can overshadow the importance of understanding and truly listening to our parents. In visiting with my senior clients, they will tell me how frustrated they are with themselves and their children. They truly love their children but are upset with their lack of understanding when it comes to the parents' emotional well-being. The older adult is facing a daunting move. The current senior generation, the seventy- to ninety-plus-year-olds, has always been fiercely independent. The thought of relying on others to make their move is distasteful at best. They know their children have busy lives and their own children to worry about. So how do both parent and child understand one another when beginning the process of moving?

Listen, listen, and listen!

If you want your parents to hear your advice, first listen to them. Intently. Quietly. Calmly. Do not rush them, just waiting for an opportunity for them to stop talking and for you to tell them what they need to do. Hear what they are saying. Understand it. Practice the effective listening skills you have heard about. Repeat back to them what you hear them saying so you and they can be sure you understand their words and intent. Ask questions about what emotions they are experiencing when thinking about the move. Find out what are their greatest fears and talk about them. Understand the memories and intangibles, such as their feelings of deep loss and sadness as they think of giving up their home. For each senior, moving elicits a different set of issues, both mentally and physically. As their child, offer support by closely listening to all that this process means to them.

When you feel you have fully absorbed their message and they also feel you have, you can have your turn. Now you can suggest solutions that take their needs and wants—and fears—into account. (I will give you more about that last one later so do not rush into it yet.)

In the end, by intensely listening to one other, each party will be more likely to work together for a positive outcome. Both parent and child will better understand the set of issues the other is facing throughout this emotional period. Together, it will be easier to obtain important information necessary for this significant moment in time. By listening to each other, a new and even stronger bond between parent and child can occur! Know that a family's love for one another will overcome the many obstacles faced when starting the process of relocating to new surroundings. Remember that, as you tread through new territory, both parent and child have one common goal—happiness and security for the older adult and peace of mind for the children!

Getting Both Parents to Communicate

Important decisions, such as moving from a long-time home, involve many different family dynamics. In addition to children dealing with their siblings and children with their parents, husbands and wives must also communicate effectively with each other.

I hear all sorts of stories at my seminars about moving for seniors. At one, a woman of a couple stood up and said that she had wanted to make a move from their home to senior housing for many years. She said that her husband sitting next to her would never leave their home. He had stated that the only way he would move was to be taken out in a box. She then proclaimed that the last time he had said that, she had told him, "When they take you out in the box, would you please take all of your junk with you?"

The audience laughed, and eventually, her husband did make the move without being put in a box. When their differences were out in the open, they found a way to resolve them.

Too often, differences between husband and wife are kept hidden.

In discussing these points, if you are dealing with both Mom and Dad, pay close attention to how each responds. Too often, I find with couples that the two partners are not on the same page. One wants to move; the other does not. Or one wants a smaller house, but the other wants senior housing. So the two avoid talking about the issue altogether. Or, when pressed by you, only one might answer. Silence by one of your parents and letting the other respond to your questions can indicate a serious disagreement on what they want to do. This will only create more problems as one parent, consciously or not, works to prevent what is not really wanted. No one wants to feel forced into any action. So from the start, make sure both parents agree completely. They may have to work their differences out on their own, but you may need first to identify where the disunity lies.

Make sure each parent responds to your questions in a clearly forceful way: "Yes" and not just "Well, maybe we should"; or "No way" rather than "Oh, I don't know." Hesitation or avoidance indicates weak spots they need to work out. Guide them into this treacherous (in their eyes) territory:

> "Dad, I see Mom really wants to move, but I'm not hearing what you want. This is a big step, and it won't work out well at all if you two don't agree. I'm not sure which is the right decision, but I do know you both need to decide on one—and the same one. Maybe you two had better talk this over some more. I'll give you time. But I'm not going to let this get swept into a corner and forgotten. I'm going to keep asking until I hear both of you give full support to a single decision."

Families have complex relationships between people who genuinely love one another and want the best for each other. Children want their parents to thrive with safety and security in mind. Parents want to remain vital and have their health needs met in a safe and secure environment. All in the family may have the same goal in mind, but each may have a differing path to get to that end result.

The bottom line is getting together and listening with open ears to one another. Start a conversation with family members today! Children of older adults should meet and discuss each other's feelings about their parent's well-being, and parents should openly share their feelings with themselves and their children. These conversations can never start too early. The most difficult moves come at a time when urgency trumps time for discussion. Crisis management does not allow for weeks or months of discussion. Decisions have to be made on the spot, and that is when relationships can truly suffer. Family unity and harmony are the goals of every child or parent, so take time out to listen and understand one another. Leave sibling rivalry to childhood memories so you can truly help your parents!

The Murray Family's Story

As with any siblings, the three of us daughters have unique personalities, talents, temperaments, and viewpoints, with an age gap of approximately five years between each of us. However, no matter what our opinions may be, we love each other and our parents dearly. Due to this love, whatever differences we experienced were resolved by our common goal of doing what was best for our parents. Because of our various talents and different distances to our parents (Barbara lives about two hours away, Susan lives nearly an hour away, and Connie lives fifteen minutes away), we each assumed different roles in our parents' lives throughout the years.

It has been hard for all of us to come to terms with the fact that they have aged to the point of moving out of the home they bought new sixty years ago—the home we grew up in, the home they valued and wanted to live in until they could no longer function on their own. It took a while for our parents to realize that time had come. Subsequently, each of us, including our parents, has put part of our lives on hold in order to accomplish the common goal of getting them settled into their new home, while letting go of the old home they loved.

During this entire process, we have told them often that we love them, and they know we are working with their best interests in mind.

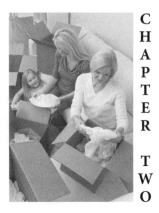

IT'S ALL IN
THE MIND

MUCH OF WHAT I suggest in this book concerns specific physical action to take—consulting experts, writing lists, tossing excess "stuff," etc. However, before your parents take any of those steps, they must have the right mindset. They must believe they are following the path that will take them to their desired goal. Without the right attitude, they will surely have a difficult journey, if they make it at all.

You may encounter much resistance in your parents considering a viewpoint other than the one they have and, possibly, have held for a long time. Fortunately, I have various methods for helping you open their minds to the many options available to them.

Changing the Story

Tony Robbins, as a guest on Oprah, expressed his frustration with the effects of his motivational workshops. His presentations get people pumped up to make changes in their lives … and then, a few days later, their enthusiasm has fizzled out, and they are doing everything just as before.

I encounter the same frustration in my talks with seniors, and I suspect you are experiencing similar feelings as you discuss options in housing with your parents.

When I speak at senior communities about a move from a long-time home to a senior community, condo, or apartment, I discuss all of the services available to make a move easy and pain-free. I give my audience countless examples of individuals in their age group (seventy to ninety-plus) who have moved successfully and are so happy they made that choice. I even have some of my past senior clients speak directly to my audience, explaining how they moved and how happy they are in their new surroundings.

After my talk, many come up to me and tell me they want me over immediately to get the process started so they, too, can make the move to their new home. They just know their life is about to change for the better!

But then, just as with Robbins's workshops, fear replaces enthusiasm from the seminar. Next, procrastination follows, and the decision to improve their lives begins to fade. The negative questions pour out, and the fire in the belly is replaced by acid indigestion. We want to protect ourselves from danger or harm, and the fight-or-flight reflex goes on autopilot. They run away from the uncertainty of a change in their lives and remain in the safety of familiar surroundings, even if that environment no longer meets their mental and physical needs.

Then they repeat a story they have told themselves for years that justifies their decision. The old story goes something like this.

> I love my home and my neighbors. It's comfortable. I've lived here for so long that this really is the only place I can call home. It's what I know, and I feel good here. Sure, the house has a few problems, but what place doesn't? I can deal with them, just as I always have all of these years.

Sound familiar? Do your parents give you a similar story whenever you try to talk about moving them to a better housing situation? Or do they agree with the idea of a move but, just like the seniors in my seminars, revert back in a few hours to staying with the same old house?

In dealing with his frustration and his audience's inevitable refusal to make the changes they supposedly want, Robbins came up with solutions. On the show, he talked about tools to create change for the better and how to make it last for a lifetime!

One tool Tony talked about was changing our story. We are often stuck in a place of frustration, sadness, or fear. Despite the negatives, the place is so familiar to us that leaving it for a better situation seems impossible. It involves negating a story that has gone on for several years, or even a lifetime. A move is just too much to take on. So, for your parents, they continue to stay in situations that are not beneficial to their mental and physical health. They know a change is needed, but they seek comfort in their current stories because they are familiar, making them feel safe, even when they know this story no longer works in their current lives.

So how can anyone overcome the propensity for staying with what is comfortable when the alternative, a change, even a small one, can enrich one's life immeasurably?

Change the story.

I gave an example of the common story I hear. What is your parents' story? Ask if you do not know it by now. Why do they remain? What reasons do they give? What excuses do they make for not considering a change? Write down what you know and have heard and even only suspect.

Then go over the story with Mom and Dad and evaluate it. Honestly. As you do, take notes for what will become their new story. Ask what is important to them and why? How independent are they in their current home? Truly. Just being in their home does not make them independent. What can they do for themselves, and what help are they getting from their children, neighbors, friends, and more? How much of their independence is "them" and how much is due to the supporting cast of people who love and help them each week? What adjustments have they had to make in their lives over the last ten years? What were they doing five to ten years ago that they cannot or do not do now? How much do they interact with their neighbors now? How difficult, expensive, annoying has maintenance of the home become?

As you discuss these questions and others related to your parents' story, a new one will begin to emerge. Write it down for them, and let them rest with it for a while.

All of us, not just our parents, often too willingly give up things in life because we think that is just life … or for our parents, it is just a part of aging. I suggest that we do not have to be quite so quick to throw in the towel and accept less out of life. Og Mandino, an author who has helped me throughout my life, said, "I can fight, rebel, resist, and even resent what is happening, or I can surrender to 'what is' and focus all of my energy on creating something better! The pain really isn't in the changes required, but in my resistance to the required changes."

Yes, it is all in the mind. Once your parents accept the idea of change—embrace it and commit to it, all else will fall into place.

Keeping an Open Attitude

In Jimmy Carter's book, *The Virtues of Aging*, he explores people's satisfaction or dissatisfaction when they reach the age of retirement. In Carter's view, we are old "when we think we are—when we accept an attitude of dormancy, dependence on others, a substantial limitation on our physical and mental activity, and restrictions on the number of people with whom we interact." His observation is that this is not tied closely to how many years we have lived.

Your parents are old in number of years, but are they old in how they think? The latter attitude has far more impact on their quality of life than how long they have lived.

In this section, I will examine our attitude, its effects upon our lives, and ways we can change it for the better. However, as much as this applies to all of us, we are really talking about the attitude of a third party, not you, not me, but Mom and Dad. We can drive them to a senior living facility and show its conveniences and explain its benefits over the situation in which they now live. But how can we get into their heads so their minds see as we do? How can we get them to change their perspective? What can we do to have them open themselves to new possibilities?

Most of you know how ineffective lectures can be—in one ear, out the other. The same applies to talking *to* our parents (actually, to anyone) when they are not ready to hear our words. So how do we get them in that ready state? Here are a few tips.

- Do not lecture. That puts you in the dominant role and places your parents in a less respectful subservient position.

- Ask gentle questions. "What do you think about …?" "Have you ever considered …?"

- Discuss friends confronting similar situations, what they did, and reasons for the outcomes they received.

- Tell stories in small doses. These are easily absorbed and remembered

Much of what follows in this chapter contains stories that encapsulate the ideas I present to you. People remember stories (and quickly forget lectures). Stories describe others, which puts a safe distance between the listeners and the action of the story. They can hear the message without feeling they must act in a certain way, as a lecture would make them feel. In time, they may feel ready to act upon the message of the story, whereas with a lecture they more likely will just deny its applicability. They reject it outright and forget it.

Take your time in discussing the issues about moving with Mom and Dad. Do not rush. And do not ram these ideas into your parents. You will only create more resistance in them. You want to create an environment that encourages communication so they hear you with open ears and an open heart.

Sprinkle stories into your general conversations with your parents. As advertisers know, we need to hear a message many times before we accept it.

Here is one story that inspires me.

We have all heard that "attitude is everything." The power of one's attitude has come into my full understanding in watching a man I knew very well coping with multiple diseases in an incredible fashion. This man was diagnosed with colon cancer, which had spread to his liver. It metastasized to other areas, including the lungs. He also was challenged with Parkinson's disease, which was first diagnosed about fifteen years before. And he had an enlarged heart, not to mention severe arthritis.

Eight years after his initial cancer diagnosis, he was still going strong! This man greeted each and every day with an incredibly positive attitude, even during chemotherapy, and went through the same rituals of showering, getting dressed, and going into the office to see what the day brought to him. This fellow Realtor loved every minute of his profession. When in the office, he went about his business of finding the best home for his clients.

He had a close family, friends, and co-workers. None ever heard any complaints about his physical condition. His number of years surviving these diseases went well beyond the doctor's predictions. "He is a walking miracle," his oncologist had said.

I know that his attitude was everything. He had said that his doctor knows his business, "but he doesn't know me!" I agree. This man was an example of wanting the most out of life and treating every day as a gift. He woke up each day with a childlike excitement as to what the day would bring. His example has forever changed my life. This man was my father.

When we approach each day with such an attitude, we leave ourselves open to see different perspectives, new opportunities, options we had formerly closed our eyes to. This is "thinking young," what Carter described in the quotation earlier.

Is that what your parents are doing? Or are they "thinking old"?

I see "thinking old" in far too many people, some with medical challenges and some in relatively good health. They are not enjoying their retirement. Instead, they are spending years in their homes in isolation. They are thinking:

- "What if I move and don't like my new home?"
- "What if the move turns into a bad mistake?"
- "How can I downsize with all of the stuff I've accumulated over the years?"
- "What if my money runs out?"

These are all understandable and legitimate concerns. In most cases, we cannot know the answers to all of our fear-based questions. But, so often, change is the best avenue for so many of our parents when confronting their housing situation. Yet they go on in isolation, living in homes that no longer meet their needs. They could be so much happier but would rather be "safe and cautious" than experience a new lifestyle that would enhance their happiness and quality of life.

Amazingly, I have yet to hear these types of questions from my seniors who are thinking about a change in their housing. Have your parents try "thinking young" with these:

- "What if I move and love the new place?"
- "What if the move gives me a more fulfilling life?"
- "What if my life will be happier with less stuff sitting around me?"
- "What if I find a way to have enough money to live happily and comfortably?"

We cannot answer these questions any better than the previous four. But they apply equally well to our parents and the thinking they must do.

Take this to heart and into your own life. Start thinking young now—before "thinking old" becomes ingrained and harder for you to change. And maybe by your doing it, you will naturally teach your parents by example.

The following advice also deals with a change in attitude, and it comes from a very smart client who told me to let others know about the "new" now. I asked him what he meant by that.

"So many seniors are resisting change and refusing to face reality," he said. "I want to make sure I get the most out of life while I am relatively healthy. For me, moving to a senior community near my home would give me that peace and security that my wife and I have worked so hard to achieve. That's my new 'now,' enjoying what I do have and not looking back."

How do your parents view their "new" now? And how do you? Do you feed their negative thinking? Do you and your parents focus on the past? Or do you and they look at the big picture, feel grateful for what you do have, and work to make now and the future the best you possibly can?

My grandmother always used to tell me, "For the same money, you can be happy!"

We have the power to decide how we want to view the world and our economy. We can look to the extremes and listen to voices of panic, or we can look to our past to help us understand our present and future. We can listen to certain radio stations and get riled up, or we can choose another station and gain a more positive attitude, remaining calm and rational. We have the power to take our remote and point to whatever cable station we choose. There have been and there always will be voices feeding fear and panic. After all, the ones that get us worked into a tizzy draw more attention than voices of calm and reason.

Consider this when talking with Mom and Dad. Where do they get their information about the world? Have they fallen into the trap of tuning into the nightly drama that features mostly negative news? They probably will not give up viewing TV, but maybe you can suggest a station with a more balanced portrayal of what is happening in our country and our world. The same applies to other sources—radio, newspapers, magazines, books. Maybe a gift subscription for them to a new publication will open a different and positive perspective for them.

Yes, the sky could fall, and the world could come to an end tomorrow, but today we can choose to focus our attention on areas we can control. Happiness and fulfillment are universal desires, so why not do all we can to experience that state of mind?

I believe in the law of attraction. What we put out into the world, either positive or negative, comes back with a vengeance. When focused on lack, we attract more of that lack and less of what we were hoping for. When we focus on fear, more insecurity comes our way. When we focus on wellness and prosperity, abundance follows. We all know folks who claim that nothing good ever comes their way and expect only bad things to happen to them. Eventually they are proved correct, confirming their announcements of doom and gloom and perpetuating their cycle of negativity.

Why not, instead, perpetuate positivity? My wife always tells me, "Thoughts become things so choose good thoughts!"

Help your parents make decisions based on a clear and positive outlook, and they will find themselves getting more out of life as well as a positive and attractive disposition!

Confronting the Options

I received a frantic call yesterday from a lovely eighty-five-year-young lady who was in desperate need of advice. She had been living in her home for the last forty years. When she had moved in, her knees were working well, and her eyesight was 20/20. She drove at night and had the home in tip-top shape. As the years went on, her husband passed away, and she was the captain in charge of the ship. She took over duties, such as paying the bills and making sure the maintenance of the home was up to the moment, as they had always taken pride in the condition, both structurally and mechanically.

Over the last ten years, her body started to experience difficulties in her ability to navigate the stairs as her knees began to show signs of arthritis. She became less confident when driving at night. And, as many of her trusted neighbors had moved, she became more anxious about security. What hurt the most was that many of her friends had moved or passed away so she became more and more isolated. Her two children lived out of town so she was alone much of the time. The home had begun to deteriorate as funds became scarcer, and the aging property had become more demanding.

Have you heard this story before? I sure have! It is heart wrenching to hear the plight of so many seniors who take pride in their homes only to be faced with a huge decision ... "Should I stay or should I move?"

I have no single, simple answer. It really depends ...

But I can offer suggestions to help you and your parents come to the best decision. Take your time to get all of the facts. Do not let fear and anxiety steal away your parents' happiness and good health. Know that their home will sell if you and they listen to the market. In the end, they can enjoy the freedoms they so richly deserve!

In the following chapters, I will help you get the facts, let you know the options available to your parents, and discuss the factors they need to consider in contemplating a move. They will need help, likely beyond what you can offer, and I will explain who can provide that. They will need to process a lot of information and much of it with emotional connections, so do not rush them. Give

Mom and Dad time to absorb the data, come to terms with reality, and make a reasoned decision that is right for them.

Your parents, and possibly you, will have a tremendous number of decisions to make. They can quickly overwhelm the best of us and push us into a defensive reaction of procrastination or avoiding the situation altogether. Do not let this happen to your parents. As I emphasize repeatedly, delaying only compounds the problem. It does not disappear but only comes back with an urgency, forcing everyone to respond immediately when fewer options will be available.

Your parents deserve better.

I will provide specific steps to take in creating a housing plan that fits your parents' needs. But first, we need to explore in more depth the current situation, what your parents feel about a possible move.

THE MURRAY FAMILY'S STORY

AFTER THEIR MOTHER had a mishap, Barbara and Dad were discussing next steps, and he said, "Well, I guess we should move now." That's when Barbara told him there were lots of available options, including revamping their home, having someone come in to clean, help cook meals, etc. When visiting a few days later, Mom looked at housing prices in the paper, and that opened the door to talk about selling and moving. She said prices were too low … but at least she was thinking about it!

At dinner that night Dad said, "All I do is sleep. I made it to ninety, so I guess it's time …," as he jokingly made a motion across his neck. Barbara asked if he had ever thought about moving to a senior retirement facility, where they play games and mingle. He replied that he would like to, "but your Ma's not very social." Despite his seeming openness to moving, Dad basically felt his life was over, that the recliner was all he had left.

In contemplating a move for their parents, Connie states, "I was more reluctant, as I had been involved in our conversations at our craft club," attended also by her mom, an aunt, and a long-time family friend. "The ladies would relay their pride at living in their homes independently; cooking, cleaning and living as they have for all of their adult lives. Additionally, I had conversations with former co-workers who had to face the same situation and knew what objections needed to be overcome. I did however realize, as my sisters did, that it would take just one slip to negatively change Mom and Dad's lives forever."

We three went to look at the actual physical locations of facilities from the outside, which helped us to eliminate several that looked good on paper and sounded good over the phone but had various drawbacks, such as a homeless person sleeping on a front-entrance bench.

Afterwards, Sandy visited Mom and Dad. They were looking over investments when the perfect opportunity to discuss the future arose. Susan says, "I told Mom, 'You and Dad have saved up a lot here. What is your goal for this?' Mom stated that she had some small savings for the grandkids and wanted to give something to her sister. She also indicated that she wanted to leave something for 'you girls' too. I asked her if they had thought any more about moving, but she stated that she was lost with all that and didn't even know where to begin. I said that we would help them and that Barbara was compiling a list of places to look at. I also stated that they really needed to strongly consider moving before something worse happened. We wanted them to move while they had the choice, rather than being forced to move later on and not being able to choose the facility."

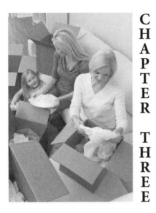

C
H
A
P
T
E
R

T
H
R
E
E

WHY MOVE?

WHY BOTHER MOVING? A house that once served your parents well may now present barriers to a comfortable life. Do any of these situations fit your parents?

- Many seniors live in a two-story home with the laundry in the basement. Yes, exercise is a good thing, but the knees are feeling the pressure of stairs, and they dread the "journey" to the second floor or basement.

- It is getting harder to navigate when taking a shower or bath.

- Driving at night is becoming an odyssey, and favorite restaurants and stores are no longer in the neighborhood.

- The home is too large, and many rooms are being used for storage facilities.

- The occupants feel like prisoners in their own home and are no longer interacting with others, instead feeling isolated.

Getting Your Parents Receptive to Considering a Move

You might think the answer to "Why move?" is obvious, but your mom and dad have likely put up all sorts of walls around the issue and refuse to see the reasons that make good sense to move. You can help them see differently by gently asking the following questions. Do not bombard them with these all at once. Instead, sprinkle them over a short time, for instance, a day's visit or several phone calls. Make some of the questions open-ended so the answers cannot get a quick and defensive yes or no. For example, instead of "Do you have problems with stairs?" which could easily get a "NO!" ask "How are you handling the stairs these days?" The latter gives a greater feeling of concern and may help them honestly consider the question—and its answer.

Here are some questions to ask your parents. They may not answer the questions—but at the least you have planted the seed to get them thinking about these issues.

- "How are you doing these days with the stairs to the basement?"
- "How is your energy level for the household tasks, especially the outside ones?"
- "Who helps you with the harder jobs?"
- "What are your feelings about living by yourself? Do you feel secure enough?" (Use if you have a parent living alone.)
- "How do you feel about driving in the dark or in adverse weather conditions?"
- "Do you have reliable contractors to make any necessary repairs or updates to your home?"
- "Are you still entertaining as you used to? What company do you have besides family?"

- "Can you properly maintain your home and make the necessary repairs and updates to keep your home in good condition?"

Maintenance of the home is the number one issue as my clients make the decision to move. It is hard to find the right help when trying to maintain the home as they would have done if health allowed. Some tasks, such as snow shoveling and yard maintenance, can be overwhelming. When you visit your mom and dad, take a hard look at their home and gently ask about significant deterioration you see, using specifics in describing the situation to them.

- "I noticed a few pieces of roof shingles on the ground after that last storm. What do you think about the condition of the roof?"
- "That crack in the basement wall seems to be getting wider. Have you noticed any leaks in it?"
- "That heavy snowfall seems to have downed a lot of big branches and even some trees. Who will help you with clean-up? Do you have anyone for pruning in the spring?"

Listing Pros and Cons

Another aid in your parents' answering why bother moving is using the "Ben Franklin list." Take a sheet of lined paper, fold it in half vertically, and at the top of the paper, put "stay" on one half and "move" on the other. Give the paper to your parents, and on the "stay" side, have them list the reasons to stay. These must be done honestly. On the "move" side, they should list all of the reasons to move. These are the quality-of-life issues mentioned, such as maintenance, stairs, etc. If they give permission, you may want to review it to make sure they have included items that you know apply.

When your parents feel they have completed it, have them put the list away. A week later, have them bring the list out, and it will talk to them. They will immediately know what is best for their individual situation. If moving looks to be the right decision for them, then it is time to gather information about the housing options available to them.

Taking Emotional Inventory

All of these questions and assessments and ideas really boil down to one question:

Is this the way your mom and dad want to spend the rest of their life?

The answer to "Why bother?" becomes, "Because I want a better life than this." Is this true for your parents? Can they honestly say that their current lifestyle is the dream they worked for their entire life? Do they want to leave their happiness to chance? If their lifestyle is right for them and the long term looks to be positive in their current home, then they can stay and enjoy their home for years to come.

Often a serious examination paints a different picture. This part of the moving process may prove the hardest for most seniors—more trying than the physical move or emotional parting. Looking closely at their life at the moment and honestly assessing shortcomings may uncover what they have been doing their best to avoid.

I call this process "taking inventory." Like any business with a stock of goods, we periodically must account for what we possess, in our case about moving, our stockpile of physical, emotional, and financial assets. What do we have, and what needs replenishing? By putting it in these terms, maybe your parents can more easily assess their situation, as if they are looking at themselves from a distance, from a business point of view.

It is a difficult task when looking at our well-being, especially as we age. We have such complex components weaving our lives together to make us who we are. As we accumulate life's many experiences, as well as mental and physical challenges, we often mask our deficiencies with self-delusion, which can lead to procrastination. At this point in their lives, your parents may have let old habits stay in place rather than change. They put off the actions needed to re-stock their physical and emotional "shelves" and often found themselves then running on empty. Therefore, when your parents do decide to begin a thorough self-examination, prepare them to face some realities that may seem a bit uncomfortable. Know that change occurs when there is some force that pushes us forward to improve our situation. When we were young, we often winged it, just reacting to obstacles in our way. Somehow, we got over them—we had to have been successful or we would not be here now. Search for examples from your own life to tell your mom and dad. Help them do the same. I am sure they can recall times that were difficult that also caused a change for the better.

In those cases, circumstances forced the change. Now, with this self-examination, your parents can drive the change. They are in charge. Focus on the positive aspects of the change and ask them, "What would it take for you to wake up each and every day with a feeling of contentment and peace? What changes do you have to make to be able to say to your friends and family that you have now reached the golden years of life and intend to stay there as long as possible?"

There is no age limit, no directional sign to the destination of happiness and contentment. It is up to each one of us to take our gift of free will and use it to our benefit. No other person can do it for us. Once your parents decide to take control of their situation and move towards a better living situation, then they may be in a position to truly enjoy their golden years.

Your parents have the power … to step into a positive and healthy new lifestyle.

THE MURRAY FAMILY STORY

CONVERSATIONS AMONG THE three of us—Barbara, Connie, and Susan—through recent years chronicled our parents' physical decline, as both parents were slowing down, losing strength, having a more difficult time with the basement steps, and in general, not being as steady on their feet causing loss of balance and on occasion tripping or "taking a tumble," as they liked to call it. They began asking for assistance with yard work and financial items, which we all gladly helped with. But we agreed that for their ages, they were doing wonderfully!

Then, in the middle of summer, we received a call from Dad saying Mom was in the hospital after falling during senior exercise class at church when her tennis shoe stuck to the floor. The diagnosis was a partially fractured femur, which would require a metal plate be attached via cables and screws. This accident and subsequent surgery was the beginning of our search for a new parental home. As we waited with Dad during surgery, we observed just how much both parents had aged, seemingly overnight. In normal day-to-day life, we had noticed small signs of slowing down, but during this stressful situation, the signs were amplified. Concern quickly increased, not only for Mom but also for Dad, who seemed to become more fragile and worn.

Barbara states, "Since I live so far away I don't visit very often, and when I do it's been sitting around the living room chatting. Though I knew my parents were aging and becoming more fragile, that did not hit me in the face until Mom fell. That's when Connie and I talked and thought we could bring services in and all would be fine, as Connie and her husband were already helping with yard work. But Susan and I also couldn't get over the one caveat … the basement. Dad used the basement bathroom almost ever since I can remember. And when Mom needed a new washer and dryer, she insisted on getting full-size replacements in the basement instead of putting stackable units in the former upstairs powder room. And not only did she use the dryer, she lugged full baskets of wet laundry upstairs to hang outside on the wash line! The basement was the nagging fear that even with help, that basement would still be where Dad headed every time he needed a restroom and where Mom eventually would feel the pull to do the laundry herself."

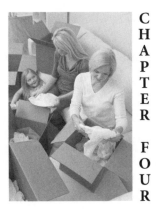

SOLVING THE UNSPOKEN PROBLEM

THE POWER TO make a change rests with your parents. But, even after listing the reasons to move and seeing the many benefits compared to staying, your parents may stall. How many times, when discussing a possible move with Mom and Dad, have they used the phrases, "I should …" or "I'm going to when …" or "I will when …" or "Maybe I'll look into …"? These words of procrastination pretend to address the situation but really put any commitments on hold indefinitely. We make excuses for not doing what our deepest sense tells us we should do primarily because of fear and anxiety.

I see another version of procrastination in my seminars for seniors—some will make a decision in their best interest and then quickly retreat. Without fail, several attendees will want me to meet with them and help them begin the process of downsizing and preparing to put the home on the market. They put a deposit down at a senior community fully intending to simplify their lives and make the move. Then hesitation sets in. Doubt and confusion begin to dominate their thoughts, and the next thing you know, they cancel the appointment and ask for the deposit back. All of this happens usually within a few days. When I speak to them after they have backed out, they express thoughts of fear and anxiety about moving, even when a move is desperately needed because of health or financial reasons.

What exactly do your parents fear about moving?

I decided to find out. I surveyed my senior clients who were still in their homes. The majority of the respondents had attended a moving seminar with information regarding affordability of senior housing, downsizing, and the process of selling their home and moving. Most of the seniors were between the ages of seventy and eighty-five years old.

Seven hundred surveys were distributed. Statistically, I expected to get back 1 percent, or seven. However, I received about 10 percent, or seventy. The questions were open-ended (subjective) with no choice of answers. The seniors were free to answer any way they chose. This was not a scientific study but simply an attempt at compiling the beliefs of seniors faced with the decision whether or not to sell their home.

What is the top fear that kept seniors from making a move?

Fear of change.

Going to new surroundings, leaving the neighborhood, and emotional separation from their home of many years were the issues on their minds when considering a move. It is hard to leave what you have known for thirty to fifty years and start over in a new home where surroundings are unfamiliar. Many of my clients had a tough time even pondering whether a move would benefit their lifestyles, despite knowing their current residence was not meeting their needs.

Too often, we know inwardly what is best for us, but we build a wall between our best intentions and our safety zone.

The best way to move your parents out of fear and towards a healing and healthy living situation is through education and helping them learn the truth about their options. As you explore the possibilities with them, keep in mind this comment I have heard from almost every senior I have helped move from a long-time home to senior living.

"I wish I had done this sooner!"

Remaining Independent

My talking and listening to many service providers of senior services, as well as seniors themselves, has confirmed that the outstanding theme running throughout the senior community regarding moving is not the sale of their home! The issues causing procrastination and hesitation are the same as they have been for many years: the fear of change and the fear of losing one's independence.

Unfortunately, too often, fear has guided seniors to communities when they have little choice—when they are near the end of their life and in poor health. The results of their delaying only confirm their worst fears: loss of independence. The frustration coming from all of us working to better the lives of seniors is that these older adults we have been talking with for months or years never have the opportunity to enjoy senior living in its best form—with independence and relative good health.

The fear of losing independence has always been at the top of the list of reasons for not making a move that ironically would provide more independence! That is at the heart of the procrastination that can frustrate all of us who truly care about improving the quality of life for our loved ones.

The Solution

Because our parents' fears often come from misperceptions or inadequate information, the best antidote for their fear that a move will strip them of their independence is to visit communities and talk to the residents, especially friends and former neighbors who have made the transition. Schedule some tours for them and let them see for themselves. Have them ask the hard questions and make sure they get specific answers. What is daily life really like in the communities they are considering?

Remember to keep good communication as the foundation of all action concerning change for them. Listen and learn about the fears, anxieties, and reasons for resisting a change for the better. Know that any change comes hard for most of us, and changing where your parents live at this stage in their life must involve overcoming not a loss of freedom but a *fear* of that loss.

We humans will go with familiarity whether it is right or wrong for our lives. Therefore, my best advice is to make the unfamiliar familiar to your parents. Help them learn the options and see what they mean in actual daily living. Tell them about seminars, which are usually free and can give a good overview of the options open to them.

Later in this book, I will go into more detail about what they can learn from professionals who can advise them. For now, know that they can find reliable information from many experts. They can talk to their financial consultants or banker to see what assets are available to sustain a monthly payment that would last them a lifetime. They can call a Senior Real Estate Specialist (SRES) to determine the current value of their home. They can visit apartments and senior communities that fit their budget. Any marketing agent within senior communities will help them understand the fees and up-front charges. They can also visit with senior planners and placement services to help them through the myriad choices currently available in their area, examine their current financial situation, and show how much it really costs them to live in their current home and maintain their current lifestyle.

If you have the time and your parents are willing, you may want to accompany them on some of these visits. Another perspective can help in remembering what was said or what questions to ask.

At their leisure, they can read books and magazines dedicated to educating so they can overcome the fear and anxiety due to lack of information. Knowledge is power, and lack of information and facts is paralyzing. How much freedom and enjoyment they have in their life is up to them.

Facing Downsizing

Your parents' trepidation about facing the inevitable changes that come with moving often center around a fear of downsizing. This one term covers many issues, which respondents in my survey mentioned: packing and sorting, giving up family treasures, starting the downsizing process, worrying about physical exertion from moving, and deciding what to do with all of their belongings. I have talked to hundreds of seniors at my seminars about all of the excess belongings they face doing something with, and downsizing hits the top in their trepidation when contemplating a move.

Obviously, the physical aspects of downsizing concern our parents as much as the emotional ones do. As their children, you can help on both fronts.

The Solution

Assure your parents that you will help them. What you offer should be realistic, given the other demands in your life. If you have the time, you can help with the sorting, packing, transporting, etc. Or you can arrange for someone else to help—outsiders for a fee or other family members. Make sure you discuss this with the others. Remember how communication is so important throughout this process. Find out who can help and in what way. And make sure your parents are included in the discussions. Do not just railroad your ideas of help into their life. These are their possessions, and they will invariably want a say in what happens to them. Include every "party of interest" in the decisions and do your best to make sure all contribute in some way—with time or resources—to keep it as equitable as possible.

When confronting the pile of possessions facing you and your parents, take baby steps. They took thirty to fifty years to accumulate their personal belongings, and they will need time to let go emotionally before letting go physically.

In Chapter 6, I give you specific steps to take in dealing with all of your parents' "stuff." Having a plan that will take care of it all, having a checklist to follow, and having people assembled to help with the various aspects of downsizing make this task feel doable. Often, not knowing where to start translates into not starting at all. With the plan, you will ensure that the job gets done and everyone survives the process healthy, satisfied, and on good terms with each other.

Dealing with Uncertainty

Our parents, like most of us, fear change, especially one as drastic as moving out of their home of umpteen years. They do have significant control over that change—they can decide where and when to move, how to handle the downsizing, what price to ask for their house, etc.—and even, whether to make the move at all.

Regardless of their decisions about the move, they have a much greater fear of the one aspect over which they have very little control: fear of the future.

The most terrifying component of the future for our parents is their health. Specifically, their greatest concerns include loss of physical ability, problems making decisions, and pain and suffering. Many also wonder about the future of their spouse if their own illness or death leaves the remaining spouse with hardship and loneliness. Some seniors worry about being left alone with no one to care for them if their spouse should become ill.

The Solution

When dealing with these issues with your parents, remember that they do have cause for concern. Do not simply dismiss them. These problems may well enter their lives, later or much sooner. For now, what can you do to help them?

First, keep communication open. Discuss their fears. Issues bothering them and kept hidden only grow in intensity. By talking with your parents, the fears lessen. Venting helps, and so does sharing problems and knowing someone else cares, understands, and is working to alleviate the worry.

Second, make sure your parents control what they can. None of us can predict our future when it comes to health issues. But we do know that exercise and proper diet can give us a better quality of life and, in many cases, extend our lives.

Third, deal with the greatest impact of all of these fears: worry. Some people will always find something to worry about, so you may have a limited opportunity to help if your parent is a born worrier. But even though the worrying concerns future uncertainties, our parents can do something to lessen the likelihood of some of those issues, such as living a life of loneliness, right now.

Get your parents connected, involved. The most active seniors are the happiest people I know. Volunteering and joining organizations can give them a sense of purpose and well-being, as well as provide a network of friends and cohorts who can be there when they need them most. By staying busy, illnesses are less frequent, and overall health is improved. Give them a nudge. Suggest places to go, societies to join, events to attend. Many nonprofit organizations need help, and feeling useful in donating time to them boosts our emotional strength tremendously. Have your parents find out what their friends do or belong to. Opportunities abound. The more time they spend participating, doing, helping, the less time they have for worrying.

Finally, help them allay real concerns that feed their fears. Listen and separate general fear of the future from specific issues, such as having adequate funds to support them in the future. And then seek sound practical advice. Certified Senior Advisors (CSAs) are available and ready to help organize your parents' financial and health needs. CSAs are trained to understand Medicare and Social Security, as well as senior housing options. They can suggest ways to extend finances and prepare for the future so your parents are not left alone or without means to deal with health and financial needs. They can look at your parents' fears and concerns and turn them into strengths and assets. Fear usually arises from lack of adequate, reliable, and relevant information.

Remember fear is False Evidence Appearing Real. Get the best information out there, and keep fear at bay.

Facing Our Feelings

Because so much about our house involves family—raising children, celebrating holidays, establishing or carrying on traditions, etc.— the story we create about our home usually includes relationships with those we love. When you went over your parents' story with them, did you see this? Did they mention the emotional connections they feel to their home because family is tied so intimately to the place?

The importance of family especially struck me after my wife and I watched *Up in the Air*, a sobering story of a man, played by George Clooney, who really had no meaningful connections with people. (You might even watch the movie with your parents to help bring out a discussion about this topic.) The man's goal was to reach the pinnacle of air travel for frequent flyers—ten million air miles. The only way to accomplish that goal would be to spend most of his life flying from one city to another. Imagine that, spending more time in the air than with family or friends. With that kind of schedule, he had no time for relationships.

After the movie, my wife and I remarked how similar the business traveler was to many of our senior clients. Like him, too many of them are isolated and lonely. Often I come home from appointments after meeting with senior clients, saddened by the lack of contact they share with others. Most have families but are disappointed that visits are infrequent due to their children's active and hectic lives. They do not want to bother their children and ask for more time with them. Many of their friends are gone, and often they do not want to leave the house if the weather is bad. The result is that they are alone for most of the time in their long-time homes.

It seems so obvious that someone in an isolated environment who wants more social interaction would choose happiness and move to a place that encourages connections with others. But human nature stops us from moving too quickly. We react to significant change with panic, confusion, and a feeling of being frozen in our tracks. As it becomes obvious that a move is the right thing to do, we get up the courage and energy to begin the process of moving. We decide to begin by downsizing. We go to our basement ready to begin, only to become overwhelmed by the enormity of the project at hand. We then walk back upstairs with hands up in the air and decide to put it off for another day. How frustrating!

The Solution

No physical barrier keeps our parents from following through. Only their thoughts, which relate to their feelings, hold them back. How they feel about leaving their long-time homes is the critical issue that must be addressed, or they will stay attached to situations much longer than they know they should.

Maybe your parents have isolated themselves so long in their home that they have forgotten how wonderful connections with friends make them feel. Open the door to talking with your mom and dad about this. Help them remember, and let them see they can form those connections again.

Do your part too. Let them share more in your family doings during this time that may be tearing at them emotionally. Just visiting your home, if you live nearby, and watching your children come and go, joining in a simple meal, watching a show together can emphasize that family will still be family, regardless of where they live. Besides getting out of their house, informal visits allow your parents to connect with those they love. Often, just "being around" allows for wonderful opportunities—normal conversations with grandchildren or catching a grandchild's first step.

If you live out of driving distance, call often to reassure them of their place in your life, in your heart. Send a card with a handwritten note now and then. Imagine how real mail stands out in the abundance of junk in our mailboxes these days. Be assured your parents will display the card as a reminder of the connection.

As your parents begin again to share their gifts of love and friendship with those who would be enriched by the connection, your parents can find new meaning and excitement in what life truly has to offer ... experiencing the joy of community. This your parents can experience once more.

TOM'S STORY

I FIND THAT men often cling most tightly to routine, to their long-time home, to situations that do not serve them but feel safe because they are familiar. Reluctant to make a necessary move, they are a bit territorial about their home and do not want to give up their cherished personal parts of the house—a garden, the man cave in the basement, a shop setup in the garage with electrical outlets and a space heater. So it was with Tom.

I met Tom after a phone call from his very frustrated wife, Cheryl, who asked for help in beginning the process of downsizing a large home and moving to a local senior community. I answered many questions but noted a frustration in her voice. I decided to wait until my appointment later that week to get past some of the surface layers of upset and uncover the main issue facing Cheryl.

As I entered their three-bedroom ranch home, I noticed Tom, bent over at a 90-degree angle, looking frail and sad and avoiding my gaze. After Cheryl gave me a great tour of their home, we sat down at their dinner table to talk. Tom proceeded to let me know that his wife was "pushing" him out of their long-time home, but I should deal with his wife, and he would "go along" with any decision she would make. We did just that—downsized and sold Tom and Cheryl's home, and they moved into a senior community near their home.

Some time passed with my hearing nothing more from them, and then I noticed a man at the YMCA. I was reading my daily newspaper while working out on an exercise bike and saw this fellow in his early eighties on the walking path, which was just in front of where I sat on my bike, moving at a rather fast pace for his age. He looked familiar, and after his third orbit on the track, I realized, to my surprise, this was Tom! I was in disbelief. This man, frail and bent over just a year ago, was briskly walking with a smile.

"Tom, it's me ... Bruce."

Tom recognized me and pulled over to talk with me and immediately apologized for his attitude during his "exile from his home."

I asked him what had triggered this transformation from a sad and frail man to the one standing tall with a smile.

He said the following. "It was difficult for me to give up my privacy and my home. I knew the neighborhood had changed—all of our friends had moved away. The stairs were killing me, and I rarely talked to anyone. But I had my workroom with all of my tools in the basement. I hadn't used that room in years, but those were my memories. My garden was unattended for many years, but that was my territory, my patch belonging to me. My health was deteriorating, and my back was causing incredible pain. Then we moved.

"About two months into my new apartment, I noticed my back pain was dissipating. I was standing straighter. I was also eating three healthy meals a day, and I felt more energy. My attitude was improving, and I met some old friends, who, to my surprise, had moved to this same community. Eating a meal with others as opposed to sporadic sit-down dinners in my old home added to my attitude adjustment.

"Now feeling better, I joined an exercise class. My health plan included a free membership to the YMCA so I decided to take advantage. I began to walk for thirty minutes a day and now up to fifty minutes! I feel better than I have felt in many years. I am enjoying every day, and my wife has a new husband. I apologized to her for my reluctance to move and my poor attitude. I let her know that her husband was back and ready to live again."

Tom readily agreed to let me share his story with others, and I thanked him.

The story of Tom is not an isolated experience. I have seen this over and over throughout my career. Change is difficult, but there is hope and life ahead if we choose to accept the necessary steps to happiness.

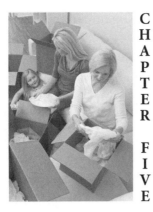

CHAPTER FIVE

CHOOSING WISELY

Now THAT WE understand both sides of the issue—reasons for your parents' staying and those for their moving from their long-time home, how do you move forward to make the best decision possible and create the best life for all involved?

Seeking Friendly Advice

When making the most important decisions of our lives, whom do we count on to give us the very best advice? Think back, look over the course of your life, and highlight the moments when decisions had to be made. This applies to you as well as to your parents. Does there seem to be a pattern as to who helped the most with the more difficult decisions you were impelled to make?

The decision to move to a new home, whether it will be a senior community, a senior apartment complex, a condominium, or another single-family home, may be one of the most difficult thought-provoking times of your parents' life. My experience in working with thousands of seniors who have lived in their homes for many years has led me to the belief that they need to consult with others who can give objective and intelligent advice when making important life-changing decisions.

When looking back, your mom and dad relied on many people for advice. Some had an agenda. Some cared about your parents, but too many past scars or negative experiences tainted the advice they gave. And some did not fully grasp the significance of the decision from your parents' perspective. But a very few always seemed to be correct in their guidance. They understood your parents, they sized up the situation, and they had that acute sense of knowing what the outcome would be. These are the people your parents need to seek out, to express their feelings and desires and wishes about a possible move to new housing.

Having established who these people, these pundits, are, your parents should write down a list of pluses and minuses for moving and the same for not moving out of their present home. (Get ideas from the "Ben Franklin list" exercise you had them do near the beginning of Chapter 2 with reasons for staying and for moving.) Have your parents call each guide and meet and discuss their lists of concerns. And then they need to ask for an opinion and write it down! It is important to see it in writing so that your parents can see exactly what their guides said. We tend to color others' opinions and remember only what matches our own. Recording the actual words keeps us honest with ourselves and helps us remember accurately.

Asking the Experts

Next come the professionals.

If you or your parents relish the idea of maintaining full control of all aspects of a possible move—investigating all options, figuring costs and fees, making assumptions about health, investments, and government assistance, etc.—then you may not need outside help. Go fly with it. Just make sure you or your parents have plenty of time, an accountant's love of detail, and the ability to work with numbers.

Most of us do not, and we will benefit from paying for the expertise of professionals. Some advice is even free.

Marketing Directors of Senior Communities

I suggest calling any senior housing community and asking for the marketing director. Most marketing directors are well versed in costs and pricing issues. There are also senior placement services that specialize in assessing individual needs (physical and financial), who will guide you to the best options to meet the demands of your parents' situation.

After your parents have determined funds available and how best to utilize them, they can go back to talk to a marketing director at a senior housing community. They will have the information necessary to discuss their options intelligently. Many wonderful communities will share their knowledge with interested parties at no cost!

Financial Advisors

CPAs and financial planners can also put fact in front of fiction. These professionals can assess your parents' entire portfolio and help you all understand where they stand financially. They can show how much your parents will have available each month for total living expenses so that they will never run out of funds.

If your parents have their own financial advisor, they should discuss this possible change with that specialist and learn what assets they will have available, when the assets will be available, what type of lifestyle their funds will support, etc. Your parents may have discussed these issues with this person before, but the sale of their home and a move to a senior housing facility, if not previously covered, will likely change advice previously given to them. Make sure your parents' financial advisor is kept informed of any significant changes in their life—health issues, sale of home, move, etc.

I find that many of my senior clients who, when they first resist the idea of moving, justify remaining in their home because it is free. In all cases, that is not reality.

With no mortgage payment, it sure seems as if living in our homes is the cheapest way to live. But we must take into account the true costs of remaining in our homes. Let us look at a few of them. A major cost is home maintenance. This includes repairing or replacing major systems, such as basement structure, roof, plumbing, furnace, and electric. Taking into account the state of these systems as they age, an unexpected bill may be on the near horizon. These upgrades or repairs can be quite substantial.

Second, property taxes and future tax increases must be paid. Included in property taxes may be current or future special assessments for street, alley, sidewalk, sewer, or water improvements.

Next, homeowner's insurance and personal property insurance must be assessed. These costs have steadily been on the rise. Claims can cause an immediate increase or rejection of policy.

Another cost of housing is the service providers your parents currently use to maintain their home. Lawn services and snow removal are constant companions. Handymen and delivery services are also needed. I hear from so many of my clients that these service providers are not always reliable or affordable. Also, consider that your parents' dependence upon such outside help will likely increase as their ability to do the physical work they once did decreases.

I work closely with senior financial planners so that my customers have all of the financial facts before making an important decision, such as moving to condominiums, apartments, or senior communities. These trained professionals will interview my clients and point out the actual costs to live in their homes, many of which I mentioned above, including utilities, taxes, insurance, and maintenance.

Most seniors understand that they will pay these costs, one way or another wherever they move. They may pay them directly as they do now in their home, or the fees may be included in an overall fee, such as homeowner's association fee for condominium owners. But if they move to a smaller home, these fees will likely be less than what your parents now pay.

However, many seniors do not realize another and more significant cost they incur by living in their long-term home—the cost of the equity in their home not working for them. Your mom and dad are living in a home that, in many cases, is a significant part of their estate. But that money just sits there. It provides a roof over their heads, yes, but by selling the house, they could buy a smaller "roof" and have money left over to invest—and have that equity work for them.

Most homeowners will pay little or no tax on capital gains when the home is sold. Couples can claim an exemption of up to $500,000 in gain, and single homeowners, up to $250,000 in gain. The requirement is to have lived in the home for two out of the last five years as the principal residence, which most of our parents have done. Therefore, when the home is sold, this tax-free equity can be invested to work for their independence and freedom.

Senior Real Estate Specialist (SRES)

Senior Real Estate Specialists (SRESs) are real estate agents that have training that focuses on the unique needs and situations of seniors looking to sell and/or purchase a new residence. Because, for over 40 percent of all older adults, their home is the largest asset in their retirement portfolio, the agent they choose will be critical to the success or failure in reaching the maximum of this asset. An SRES will design a comprehensive plan to meet your parents' specific situation.

Your mom and dad may have received well-intentioned advice from many people about selling a home. How much of it is true?

The SRES can discuss the issues and separate any rumors Mom and Dad may have heard from the facts. In addition, a seasoned agent can bring the entire downsizing, moving, and selling processes to a smooth and successful conclusion. Think of this professional as your most valued partner as you guide your parents to their new home.

Before interviewing and committing to a specific Realtor (which I address in Chapter 8), have your parents, possibly with you, talk to a real estate agent, preferably an SRES, to get a feel for how much their house is worth. Have them ask about fees they can expect to pay, and listen to what the agent suggests for improvements to the home.

Your parents are doing just preliminary work at this point, laying the foundation for what will follow.

Attorneys

Your parents will also need to know how these changes will affect their estate, which will change throughout their lives, impacted by both their finances and health. An elder law attorney has the knowledge and expertise to guide your family through the maze of the many legal issues related to their estate and taxes. I encourage you to seek out a good elder law attorney early in the process. This will ensure that they are able to make informed decisions that will positively impact their future well-being.

Movers

In contemplating the physical move, your mom and dad will want to know the costs of moving their possessions. There is an organization called National Association of Senior Move Managers (NASMM) that will likely have members in your community. A moving consultant can explain all of the services available for downsizing, packing, and moving your parents' personal belongings to their new home.

Summary

When your parents speak with the professionals, you may want to accompany them. An extra ear to hear and remember the advice given in these meetings serves everyone well. You can also make sure certain questions are asked and the answers understood. In my survey of seniors and professionals serving them, all mentioned that cost was the most confusing when contemplating a move to senior housing. This included differences in prices, cost increases, affordability on a fixed income, entry fees, and payment plans.

In summary, here is a list of professionals your parents may wish to include when seeking advice:

Marketing Directors of Senior Communities
Financial consultants
    CPA
    Financial planner
    Certified Senior Advisor
    Senior financial consultant
    Parents' own financial advisor
Senior Real Estate Specialist (SRES)
Attorney
Moving consultant (NASMM)

Looking at Housing Options

Your parents probably have many thoughts about what a new home would look like, its location, and the services it offers. Before taking any tours, organize those ideas. Once more, have your parents put pen to paper and write down their feelings, thoughts, and desires. What do they want, or what might they want? What elements are important to them? Also, what do they not want in their new home (such as stairs or changes in floor levels)? They may feel they cannot have everything they desire, but that constraint does not enter the picture now. They should list all that they really want and prioritize them. Each entry need not have a number assigned to it. Instead, they may want to group items:

- absolutely must have
- definitely want
- would be nice
- only if funds permit.

They may want to alter their list once they see more housing situations. Tours of actual layouts may give more ideas about what works well, what especially appeals, and what arrangements would be desirable that they had not even thought about. Putting these ideas in written form enables our goals and needs to become real. They become tangible and more likely to come about in physical form.

Start them thinking about location. You have heard the phrase, "location, location, location" when talking about real estate sales and values. It applies equally to where your parents will live. This factor is so vital to their happiness and comfort. Maybe your parents already have a general area in mind. Or you may have to drive them around to expose them to the possibilities. If your parents' health allows them to live independently, check out the layout, services, and amenities offered, whether people are out and about, and your gut feeling when you walk in. If their health is compromised and decisions are left up to you, location and aesthetics are important, but more critical are the level and quality of care. Once they have the location narrowed down, you can help them investigate the types of living situations available in the area.

Meanwhile, to help your mom and dad adjust to moving to that locale, suggest they visualize themselves in it. How does it feel when they drive home or walk out the front door? Are their doctors, restaurants, children, friends, and favorite stores close to their new home? They may not find all they desire, but they can have the ideal in mind against which to compare the places they look at. Then they can judge how close they come to finding a new place that includes as many of the important people and places dear to their heart.

Your parents now have a good idea of the general area they want to live in. (By the way, a majority of people who move stay within a few miles of their long-time home.) Exactly what housing options exist there? And how do they compare to each other? Here are the general types of living situations your parents might consider.

Condominium

Condominiums are typically purchased just like single-family homes. They are set up as a complex of units. There are many variations of the types of condos available. Some are side-by-side ranch units with attached garages, and others are among several units in a building with an elevator and underground parking. A condo fee, usually assessed monthly, covers maintenance (short- and long-term) of the buildings and grounds. The price depends on the location, as well as square footage of each unit. The outside maintenance is usually handled by the condo fee. Improvements needed can be assessed to each owner, although there is typically a reserve fund for such repairs. A call to your Senior Real Estate Specialist can get you more specific information on fees and what they cover.

Senior Apartment Complex

A senior apartment complex is a group of apartments that cater exclusively to older adults. Individuals must be able to care for themselves and will find limited services available.

Retirement Community

A retirement community is a self-contained residential development designed for older adults. Support services and recreational and social amenities are often available.

Continuing Care Retirement Community

A continuing care retirement community offers three levels of living:

1. Independent

2. Assisted living (which includes community-based residential facilities, or CBRFs, and residential care apartment complexes, or RCACs); see "Assisted Living" below.

3. Skilled nursing facility, or SNF (which includes nursing home and health centers)

The individual moves from one level of care to another, and sometimes from one housing unit to another, as needs change. Having these various levels of service within one community ensures continuity of care as health changes occur.

Life Care Retirement Community

A life-care retirement community is similar to a continuing care retirement community but is distinctive in two ways:

1. It requires payment of an endowment/entrance fee. This fee has very limited refundability and is intended to cover some of the expenses for the individual's future care.

2. The individual has guaranteed placement in their skilled nursing facility.

Assisted Living

Each state has laws that regulate and define this type of housing. The following is general information.

1. Residential Care Apartment Complex (RCAC)

2. Available services include personalized assistance with activities of daily living and health care. Supportive services range from minimal to a very high level of assistance. These facilities must be registered with the state.

3. Community Based Residential Facility (CBRF)

4. CBRFs are state-licensed and regulated facilities that are staffed twenty-four hours a day and provide personal assistance, help with medications, supervision, and three meals a day. Admittance is based on the residents' ability to ambulate, follow directions, and act for self-preservation under emergency conditions.

5. Adult Family Home

6. This is a facility serving four or fewer residents.

To get a feel for what these descriptions mean in actuality, your parents need to visit them. Maybe they have friends now living in some and can visit and get an insider's view. Or perhaps you will play chauffeur for them as they get an intimate look at a possible home. As you tour communities, you will be able to gather pricing information and begin to make comparisons.

Once your parents have narrowed down the choices, revisit their selections with a trusted advisor to get their perspective and input. Each step along the way of selecting possible housing arrangements narrows the choice—to a specific area, to a specific type of facility, to one or a few specific facilities or homes. Each round requires decisions. Facts may support one choice over another, but one of the best guides for making a sound selection is, as before, your parents' inner voice, their gut feeling.

The most successful moves I have been a part of involve clients who have done sufficient planning, who have researched and visited the choices available, and who know what they want. "Know thyself" is a phrase most appropriate to finding the right place to live.

THE MURRAY FAMILY'S STORY

WHILE MOM WAS still in the hospital recovering from her surgery, Barbara called the Milwaukee County Commission on Aging/Resource Center. They mailed a large catalog containing senior living options ranging from independent living to continuing care. Barbara focused on independent living, narrowing it down to twenty options. Subsequently, she spoke with management at each facility asking the same questions. Each family's criteria will be different, but this was ours:

- Location – Only those facilities that were in their current area and close to their church, a very important part of their lives.

- Size – The larger the facility, the more options for activity would likely be offered, yielding more opportunity to make friends with similar personalities.

- Meals – Mom still cooked so they would not use the Senior Center meals. To provide a broad range of choices, facilities with no meals, with meals, and with minimum meals that could be increased in the future were all included. The food had to be good if they were going to be "stuck" with it, which was brought up in the interview process.

- Unit Sizes/Bathrooms/Balcony – Some were eliminated from the list because they only had two bedroom/one bath, which would not work for our parents. It was important that they be able to step outside and get a breath of fresh air, so a balcony option needed to be offered. (Ultimately, they chose an apartment without a balcony.)

- Cost – Endowment facilities were eliminated as well as those with "continuing care." Reduced and subsidized rentals were investigated, and it was found that the reduction was not uniform but, rather, based upon outside factors. All pricing was written down as our parents' exact financial situation had not yet been finalized.

- Activities – Enough offerings to interest both parents. While a pool table would be top on the list for Dad, Mom would prefer a crafting get-together. While most places offered bingo, that did not interest them.

- Extras/Services – Our parents still drive, but what about when they can't anymore? Did the facility provide transportation to the grocery store? The mall? Did a hairdresser visit the facility? What about clergy or church services? Was there onsite banking? Is there anything else that the facility manager felt was of importance?

- Affiliation – Are they affiliated with an assisted living/ongoing care facility if Mom and Dad needed more care, or what options were available?

- Parking/Utilities – Some included parking, others charged. Same with utilities. These charges needed to be included in monthly budgets, no matter how small the fee might be.

Barbara then made a list of the top ten and developed detailed data sheets to help compare the facilities and highlight their offerings. Barbara finalized facility information and set up tour appointments with the facilities we had picked. Based upon what Mom had said about waiting a couple of weeks and not being ready to move yet, just the three of us were going to go on the tours. But after further thought, we felt it would be best to involve Mom and Dad from the beginning, if they would agree. That was the really hard part—telling them that we had moved forward and made appointments! After some discussion, it was decided that since Barbara had done the research and made the appointments, she would let them know about the appointments and invite them to come along. We hoped they would agree. Barbara called them the day before and told them she had something important to talk to them about … that we had appointments to look at some senior residential facilities and would like them to go, too. This was extremely difficult for Barbara to do as none of us knew what their response would be! Mom agreed they would tour, though "We're not at the point of moving yet."

After the first day of apartment visits, Mom became more interested and stated that she would like to visit some place with graduated care and meal options. We visited assisted living facilities that were adjacent to two of the senior apartments we had looked at, but one was more like a nursing home (depressing) and the other was cost prohibitive.

During the second day of visits, one complex won them over. It was in a great location and had a bright cheery central lounge area with high ceilings and lots of windows, and we were able to eat lunch there, which we all agreed was very good. They were very pleased with the facility, so they agreed to be placed on a waiting list! Mom's physical therapist echoed us on the move, saying it was better this way that they choose the place now, while they could.

At the same time, Susan did a number of detailed budgets for Mom who was concerned about being able to afford the apartment. Even though there would be a deficit every month, they would be able to draw on savings until their IRA distributions came at the end of the year, at which time they could replenish their savings. She also ran a number of worst-case scenarios and helped Mom see that it would all be okay in the end, even if they had to eventually go into the skilled nursing facility.

Susan had also suggested their parents see an Estate Planning attorney that specialized in Elder Law in order to be sure their wills were updated, trusts were setup, and healthcare and financial power of attorneys in good form. Her mother indicated they were not ready to move yet but agreed on seeing the attorney as she knew it was time to do the proper planning (which included pre-planning and paying for their funerals).

After several meetings with the Estate Planning attorney, everything was set up properly, and the plan was put into place. On one hand, this was an emotionally stressful time for them as it meant change, but on the other hand, it was a huge relief to know that the financial decisions that were made would allow them to accomplish their current and future goals. The attorney we had was wonderful! She was patient, kind, compassionate, thorough, and fair. She really took her time, answered questions, and put our parents at ease throughout the whole process.

It cannot be stressed enough what an important role an experienced Estate Planning attorney plays in the process, preferably one that specialized in Elder Law. Proper planning before moving is an essential step that provides tremendous relief in the end.

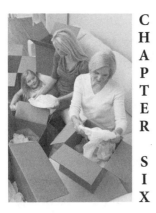

C
H
A
P
T
E
R

S
I
X

CREATING THE HOUSING PLAN

What Do Your Parents Really Want?

As I enter into a conversation with my clients, I ask, "How motivated are you to make the move into a new home? Why are you considering moving?" It is critical to establish the urgency to make a move. Making a move from any home is a highly important and stressful decision. If motivation is weak, then I find that homeowners will subconsciously sabotage any potential sale by overpricing the home, not preparing the home properly to have a chance of attracting an offer, missing important deadlines, etc. Without a compelling reason to move, they may become angered and frustrated by the entire process and direct those negative emotions towards not only you but also the professionals they have hired to help. Deep down, we all dread change and will try to avoid that uncomfortable feeling if at all possible.

However, I have found that when we look to the future and see a better situation that will enhance the quality of our life, then we make intelligent decisions now, based on reality. A well-thought-out move will almost always be successful. Once a decision has been made to move with a strong motivation, all seems to fall in place with an appropriate plan. When I discuss price or updating the home or timing of the sale, I am working with individuals who have the same goal that I do—the successful sale of their home. I suggest they listen and think, and we come to an agreement. If we disagree, we work out the problem. We are working together as a team.

The goal is to have your parents behind their decision and highly motivated to go on. And what exactly is their decision?

Once your parents know how much money they will have available and have assembled and talked to their team of experts and advisors, they need to decide what they want. What factors matter to them, in general and specifically? How do they compare to each other? What are the priorities?

Most seniors place a high value on independence and not relying upon others for financial support. As they age, financial security becomes a greater and greater issue as their earning power diminishes. In trying to protect themselves from insecurity, many times, they overestimate what will be necessary to maintain their current and future lifestyles. Obviously, in many cases, it may be necessary to rely on others for daily living, but I am referring to those who weigh decisions far too heavily on that security and shut off the possibilities for true happiness. I have far too many clients living a life of seclusion and just trying to get by each day. When we talk about their options, many will not even count the sale of their home as an asset factor in their decision-making. I have worked with folks in their nineties who feel they need enough financial backing for the next twenty-five years! I can understand where that thinking comes from, as we want to make sure we can weather any storm coming our way, and we want to leave a legacy for those we love.

Security is certainly critical and of utmost importance when considering a transition to new housing. However, a more balanced approach between security and quality of life will provide a better outcome.

A Housing Plan

"I want to sell my home, but I just don't know when—or where—to start the process." I hear this often from my senior clients, and my answer is the same … It is never too soon to start the planning and preparation for the move. If your parents are thinking of moving in the next three to six months, now is the time to begin downsizing, making calls to professionals, and making decisions about the right housing to meet their needs.

How to begin?

They need a plan.

We have an insurance plan, we have a financial plan, but how many of us have a housing plan? Yes, a housing plan! At my seminars for seniors, I have asked this question to hundreds of senior homeowners, and invariably the response is a blank stare. We leave one of the most important aspects of our lives to chance. We wait for circumstances to dictate when we will make our next move. Unfortunately, circumstances can change quickly in the form of health changes or financial loss. It would be a blessing if we could predict the precise moment when and if these changes would occur.

But we do not have the gift of seeing the future, and we must plan accordingly.

If a catastrophic event forces your mom and dad into an immediate sale and move, with a housing plan, you all are set. Necessary improvements have been made, your parents have a Realtor on file, they know the true value of the home, and they have started downsizing or, at least, have listed what items will go with them, go to selected individuals or charities, or be disposed of. That is the essence of a housing plan.

If disaster never does strike, they will be that much better prepared for a move with them in control and the major concerns already addressed.

In the following chapters, I will describe in detail the steps you and your parents need to take to create a housing plan. They include:

- Downsizing

- Finding a Realtor

- Knowing the value of the home, based on its condition

- Improving the condition of the house

- Timing the sale

Although I focus on these steps with the idea of your parents enacting them soon, their immediately putting the house up for sale is not the only purpose. Instead, this information can be gathered and held until your parents are ready to sell. The main purpose of their housing plan is to make sure they are ready when they do want to sell. It puts them in control, which is where they want to be.

As I have mentioned before, operating in a crisis situation where you have very little time to make life-altering decisions causes stress for everyone and, often, a less-than-optimal choice for your parents. You do not want this to happen to you, nor do your parents want to burden you or any of their children with having to cope with that. This problem worsens when conditions in the real estate market work against your parents' need to sell now.

Your parents have spent countless hours planning their finances and health plans. Now they need to spend some time developing a housing plan, based on their honest needs, both present and future.

Details of the Housing Plan

If your parents have started the downsizing before they have to move, congratulations to all. They are ahead of the game.

But at some point, your parents will have a deadline to meet. Their Senior Real Estate Specialist or Realtor can give them a timeline for all of the steps that they must take in the sale of their house. If they have developed their housing plan well in advance of their need to move, they can address these points in a leisurely fashion.

To keep track of all, have your parents prepare, as here, a single list of all of the steps they must take with a must-begin and must-end date for each. Then as they complete each task, they can check it off, which will give them a sense of accomplishment and getting closer to their goal of moving into a new home.

Before Selling the Home

- Interview three real estate agents, including at least one Senior Real Estate Specialist

- Choose one real estate agent

- Have the agent inspect the home

- Meet with the agent and receive the agent's recommendation for work to be done and approximate value of the home

- Consult with a stager (if your goal is to get top dollar)

- Have professional contractors inspect the house to learn what structural issues must be addressed

- Decide what work will be done on the house

- Get bids from three companies for each project, then select a company for each project, and set dates to begin work. Start with the most important and/or time-consuming projects.
    Structural issues
    Roof

> Basement
> Furnace
> Electric
> Plumbing
> Remodeling
> Painting
> > Interior
> > Exterior
> Carpeting
> Refinishing floors
> Landscaping

- Begin downsizing
  Note what will happen with each item (sell, give, toss, or keep)
  Distribute donated items to individuals or charities
  Toss unwanted items
- Arrange estate sale (can be done before or after the home is sold)
  Interview two or three companies
  Select one
  Set date, sign contract
  Have sale (may be before or after the house goes on the market)
- Move excess possessions out of the house
- Arrange furniture and items that will stay during display of home
- Have agent do final inspection

Putting the Home on the Market

- Sign contract with agent; set asking price and date for putting the house on the market
- Photograph home (agent will likely arrange)
- Write description of house (agent will likely do with input and okay from owner)
- Schedule open houses for other agents, neighbors, the

general public

- Clean house, mow lawn, shovel snow, etc.
- Put up for-sale sign
- Put house on the market, put flyers in box on for-sale sign, post information online

WHEW!

Yes, the list is long. This is why a well-thought-out housing plan begins months before a home goes up for sale.

Regardless of how much time your parents have before selling their house, they should take it one step at a time to keep the process from overwhelming them. The same goes for you since you will invariably be involved in many of the above steps. Creating a list of steps your parents must take with the relevant dates gives structure to a task—moving—that otherwise seems huge, unmanageable, and impossible to get done in time. Not everyone will take all of these steps. For instance, your parents may choose not to engage a stager, or they may handle the sale of their items themselves. And your parents may have other jobs to add to this.

In any case, the sooner your parents start, the better for everyone.

Summary

As your parents consider the options open to them and the choices they must make, have them talk to others and learn what they think of the moves they made. I am guessing your parents will hear results similar to what I have found in my survey, as well as in my one-on-one discussions with seniors.

Of the respondents to my survey, 76 percent relayed positive statements they had heard from their friends and relatives who had made a move to senior housing. An overwhelming majority were extremely happy they had made the move from their long-time home to a senior community. Some of the statements elaborating their answers included:

- Moving gave me relief from duties at home.
- Lifestyle improved.
- I made many new friends.
- Chores and meals were prepared.
- I have travel and fun without worrying about the home.
- I should have done it sooner!

Of the 12 percent in my survey who were not satisfied and the 12 percent unsure or with no opinion about the move, several mentioned dissatisfaction because circumstances had forced their decision. That is the hardest situation to go through, both for me as a professional and for those experiencing the dilemma of a health or financial downturn. Waiting too long to make a move is so sad because, in most cases, the move could have been made when their health situation was manageable. Financial decisions, such as selling the home to free up a rather significant asset, could have been done while they were independent and in a healthy condition, physically and financially. Even more heartbreaking is watching the children or caregivers making decisions for seniors who are no longer in control of their moving situation. Why wait for circumstances to make such an important decision when they could enjoy and be active participants in a move to better their situation, both physically and financially?

Do what you can to make sure your parents do not fall into that predicament. Explore options now while they have time. Follow the steps I have outlined in making wise choices and creating the housing plan to move them out of procrastination and into action. Have your parents:

- Talk to the professionals to assess your parents' financial situation.

- Tour senior housing to get a feel for what they like and want.

- Gather information from others.

- Think about what they really want and what will bring joy to their lives.

- Assess their needs and try to anticipate future ones.

- Realistically evaluate the advantages and disadvantages of their current home.

- Take time to let it all sink in.

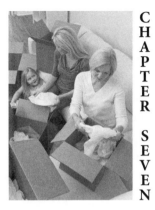

DOWNSIZING

BECAUSE DEALING WITH downsizing can seem overwhelming, in Chapter 3, "Solving the Unspoken Problem," I had you assure your parents that they will have the necessary help for this aspect of moving to a new home. As with any big job, the more hands helping, the easier the work.

Letting Go Emotionally

First, your mom and dad should assess the reality of their situation and take a good look at the space they currently utilize. I find that many seniors are occupying only a few areas of the home a majority of the time. For instance, if you measure the square footage of the areas your parents are using, it will be far less than the total size of their home. It may include only a family room, kitchen, bath, and bedroom. The formal living room, formal dining room, extra bedrooms and bathrooms, and basement rec room are all excess, hardly used. When you add up the square footage of the main living area, it may total less than eight hundred square feet! This is shocking because the total square footage of their home may be twenty-four hundred square feet or more. Now, look at the new place they plan to move into. Though it may be less than their current home, it will likely serve them better in floor plan and utility. So they actually gain living space, as well as a floor plan that better meets their needs. They will not have excess space, rooms that they hardly use, and the ones that they will use occupy more square footage than their current true living space. It all depends upon how you look at the situation.

With this new perspective, your parents may feel better about downsizing, as well as the move itself.

So many of my senior clients feel overwhelmed just at the thought of tackling this task that they put it off indefinitely, as if ignoring it will make the problem go away. But it does not. Eventually, the date of a move is upon them, and then they must rush to decide what to do with all of their possessions. Avoiding downsizing only compounds the problem. It has not gone away or diminished in size in the period of procrastination, and now with very little time to toss, give away, or move every single item in their home, these seniors *will be* overwhelmed.

Do not let this happen to your mom and dad.

My advice is to take on the downsizing bit by bit. Your parents can handle one room or one closet at a time. The whole house will definitely overwhelm them. If they tell themselves that they are doing only one part at a time, they can mentally ignore the rest, and the one section of the house seems doable.

Best of all, have them start the process now, regardless of where they are in looking for a new place to live. The more they do sooner, before the crunch of "right now," the easier the moving process will be for them when it does come. And they will have the advantage of a less cluttered home in the meantime.

Associated with the willingness to do the physical job is the permission your parents must give to releasing some of their possessions. They must let go emotionally. Are your parents ready to part with some—or even many—of their treasures? They will need to make up their minds to let go of items they have been holding onto for many years. Knowing that family or friends will take care of cherished treasures may soften the task of parting with them. And donating some of their possessions to people who have greater needs may even bring good feelings to letting go.

Once your parents feel emotionally ready to let some of their items go to new owners, you need to address the specifics of downsizing.

Sorting

As your mom and dad sit comfortably in their home, their treasures, acquisitions, and belongings surround them. Will all of these items fit in their new location? Most likely not. That leads to their next question.

"What am I going to do with all of the stuff?"

Your parents must decide what, in general, they will do with their items. Will they have an estate sale? Will they throw anything out? Consider categorizing them:

- Definitely keep and take to new home
  Items your parents absolutely need to take with them, ones they know will fit in any apartment, and things they will not part with.

- Maybe keep and take to new home
  What they might take with them depending on the size of the new home. Since it is possible they will not know the exact square footage of their new condominium or apartment, they might not want to give final say as to where these items will go until they find a new residence.

- Get rid of
Items your parents absolutely do not want under any circumstances. Put these in writing (definitely on the computer to make sharing by email fast and simple).
    o   Give to specific individuals (family, friends, neighbors, etc.)
    o   Sell
    o   Donate
    o   Throw out

What category will each fall into? They will need to assign every item they own to one of those categories. In the next section, Distributing Possessions, I will show you a relatively simple way to do this. For now, just help your parents understand what each category includes to get them thinking about what item will fall into which group.

Distributing Possessions

When your mom and dad have their list of what they will get rid of in some way, they must decide where these items will go—to whom or to where. Most likely, they will want family members to have first dibs, so alert them first. Figure out a fair way to distribute them. You want this to go smoothly for your parents and without quarrels. Let a lottery decide who goes first (for example, pick a card from a deck; lowest goes first). You can go in rounds, each person selecting one item in turn. Or your mom and dad may want certain items to go to specific individuals, maybe even outside the close family circle. Make sure you listen to and honor their wishes.

Once family has been taken care of, send the list farther afield to friends, neighbors, co-workers, other relatives, and members of your parents' church or temple. Let these people know which items your parents may want to part with and the items they absolutely do not want to keep. You may want to include items from the second category as ones that might be available, depending … Put a deadline or final date they can claim these items with your mom and dad as the contact (unless you all agree to another person handing out the items). Let the people know that if they do not respond by the deadline, these items will be donated to Goodwill or some other organization.

Among the third category, "get rid of," your parents may have valuable property that they can sell to the public. But first, make sure family knows what is going on. You do not want Mom or Dad to hear later that so-and-so had always wanted Grandma's rocking chair that was sold. Or maybe they will need the money (or, even, want to avoid sibling squabbling) so want to sell all of the items not needed for the new place. These are their possessions, and they have full rights to determine what happens to them. Again, respect their wishes. And remember to keep this an open discussion. Hiding what is going on will only hurt someone later.

If they do want to sell to the public, reputable estate-sale liquidators can handle the task. Either these companies will buy the personal property, take all to their showroom, and sell, or they will hold an estate sale at your parents' home. The general rule is that the items should be worth more than three to four thousand dollars for most companies to get involved. Their fee is generally 33–40 percent of the gross dollars brought in at the sale. The sale usually runs for three to four days, with each day discounting items, until everything is sold. The companies will typically clean the home after the sale so, with the right timing, the buyer of the home can move right in.

Whenever selecting any contractor or service, a referral is important. Therefore, ask and have your mom and dad ask friends or relatives for names of businesses they have used to help dispose of their personal property.

I have found Post-It notes to help tremendously in this process. Get a mega stack of different colors of Post-Its and have your mom and dad designate one color for each of the categories above and write down what each color stands for. For example:

- Green – definitely take to new home.

- Blue – maybe take to new home. If your parents learn they cannot take a "blue" item (because, for example, it will not fit in their new home), what will they want done with this? They will have two Post-Its for each item in this category. Blue indicates maybe the item will go with them; the second color indicates where it will go if it cannot go with them.

- Yellow – give to specific individuals. They should write on the Post-It the name of the person they want the item to go to.

- Red – sell.

- Orange – donate.

- Pink – throw out.

Then suggest your parents start with a closet or small room and attach a Post-It to each item. I would not even bother with a label for the "throw-out" items. Instead, your mom and dad can use an old cardboard box and, as they come across a throw-out item, do just that—toss it into the box. They will have less to do later, and spreading out the tossing will not overwhelm their garbage cans.

For the items to give to individuals, they may not know who should get what. And they may unknowingly want to give things to people who have no desire for them. They think others will appreciate their treasures, but how do they know for sure?

A great misconception your parents likely hold is believing their loved ones will want to have a piece of their family history or personal property that was so meaningful to them. The following story illustrates the danger of such an assumption.

A senior mother saved decorative plates. Each month, she would give away one plate to each of her two sons. She wanted to enjoy the giving and see the expressions of joy when they received her precious gift. One day, she called one of her sons to inform him she would be giving him the pride of her collection this month. She was so excited! Her son was at work when she called. He had to put her on hold for a moment, but he forgot to press the hold button. As she patiently waited on "hold," she heard every word that he said to his brother who was with him. "Hey Bill," the first son said to his brother, "Mom is on the phone, and she has more junk for us."

This well-intending woman was surprised, but fortunately, she found humor in the situation and made changes in the distribution of her "junk."

The moral of this story is that your mom and dad may think they know what family or friends would be happy to receive, but in most cases, the givers miss the mark. Family and friends will not want to disappoint anyone when they receive your parents' treasures and, so, will graciously accept them. It makes much more sense for your parents to make a list of items they want to give away and send this list to all with whom they want to share.

This process of giving to family and friends can start any time. Your mom and dad need not wait until an imminent move hangs over them. With good planning and starting well before they need to get it done, they can spread out the joy of sharing. And they can …

> Do their givin' while they're livin'
> so they're knowin' where it's goin'!

Using Professionals

If your parents have decided to sell items, they must decide whether to do it themselves or hire a professional. The choice has the usual considerations: more work for them if they do it themselves or more expense if they hire someone to do it. However, they may net more money in the end from using those who do this as a business. They know how to price items since they have more experience and familiarity with what buyers are willing to pay; they take into account inevitable bargaining; and they know how, when, and where to advertise to bring in people who will buy.

Before deciding on what route to take with selling, your parents may want to have a professional appraiser price items they plan to sell. Many of their belongings may have little to no value in today's market, but some items may be of great value when appraised by a professional. For instance, here is a list of items that will bring the most money at an estate sale or auction:

- gold, jewelry, gemstones, ivory pieces
- oil paintings, watercolors, and other art by well-known artists; antique posters
- antique furniture
- figurines, bronzes, brass, pewter, silver, china, glassware, crystal stemware, vases, clocks, sterling flatware, sterling serving pieces, silver-anything, mirrors
- antique dolls, toys, games, and lamps; model cars
- World War I and World War II items

Other items that may have value include:

- furniture, including: sofas, love seats, chairs, recliners, tables, cocktail and end tables, table and floor lamps, pianos, card table and chairs, outdoor furniture
- antique jewelry, all costume jewelry
- power tools, hand tools

More general items that will likely have less value include:

- books, both hard cover and paperback
- cookbooks

- records, cassette tapes, eight-track tapes, CDs, videos, radios, telephones
- picture frames
- bar items, fireplace tools and screen
- candles, plants, planters, floral arrangements
- sewing machines, fabrics, yarn
- office supplies, old pens, paper goods, gift-wrap items
- perfume, new cosmetics
- umbrellas

Ask family, trusted advisors, friends, and co-workers to see if they have used the services of an appraiser for any items of value and would recommend that person. If no one has referrals, then search online for a local appraiser and pay attention to the reviews. (If your parents are comfortable using the computer for this, they certainly can do it themselves.) Take great care to check out the credentials of such appraisal services. You can also refer to the Better Business Bureau in your area to make sure an appraiser you consider is trustworthy.

Your mom and dad should schedule two or three appraisers to come to their home. Make sure the appraisers know one or two others will also be bidding on the job to ensure you get fair estimates from all.

In many cases, information from the appraisers will indicate that your parents' personal property will not have enough monetary value for an estate-sale company to take on the job of liquidating their items.

You and your parents can again ask around for those who have used the services of companies that purchase used furniture. There are companies that will purchase every item you have and pay cash. Check online. If your parents or another family member has the time and energy, someone can also post items for sale on Craigslist for those items with a higher value. Look also for consignment shops in the area.

If your parents want to donate, some organizations will pick up much of their personal property as donations. In my area, for example, an organization helps battered women who need to start over in a new home setting and accepts donations of furniture, dishes, linens, etc. For a list of organizations looking for donations of this type, you can check the Internet or your parents' church, temple, or synagogue.

Handling the Physical Job

The downsizing process involves much physical work—lifting and moving boxes, furniture, and other heavy items into and out of vehicles up and down stairs. Your independent parents may want to tackle these tasks themselves. Do they have the time, a lot of time? Do they have the strength to do this for days on end? Take an honest look at their limitations, both physically and mentally. Ask them, "Can you stand on a ladder with balance? Can you stand for long periods without pain? Do you have breathing problems? Can you negotiate stairs with ease? How about when carrying a heavy box? Can you lift bulky items easily from the floor?"

Many of my senior clients have always done "it" themselves. By "it," I mean just about every aspect of their lives. Many who suffered through the Depression years learned to survive by being self-sufficient. Not only did that save money, but it also gave dignity and self-worth to many who had little else as they were losing their money and homes during those difficult years. Unfortunately, this practice can become a health risk, both mentally and physically, as constraints due to age overtake the will to accomplish formerly doable tasks.

I recently had clients who had saved an enormous number of "treasures" over the forty-five years they had lived in their home. Their health was failing, and they decided to move into a senior apartment. When I first visited with them, I suggested we get outside service companies to help with the tremendous downsizing project. There are reputable companies who specialize in organizing, packing, selling, and moving the personal property. Both husband and wife thanked me and decided to go it alone.

The process nearly hospitalized both of them. As they tried to take on the work that was beyond them, they became angry and upset at the prospect of moving. Both developed serious back problems as well as depression during the move. They would not accept anyone's help. They turned down offers from their children to assist with the downsizing. "We've never put a burden on our children, and we're not about to start now!" they adamantly stated.

The result was that this wonderful happy couple slowly evolved into negativity. They resented the buyers for forcing them into such a negative situation and became difficult to deal with when negotiating the sale of their home. What could have been a relatively easy and smooth process became the worst nightmare of their lives.

Make sure your mom and dad honestly answer those questions assessing their ability and willingness to tackle the physical move. Then you all will know whether they can handle the sorting, packing, disposing, and moving of their possessions themselves or if they will need help. Let these independent spirits know that it is okay to accept help, that, just maybe, they *should* get help.

My best advice to your parents is:

Never say no when anyone offers to help in downsizing.

When family or friends ask if they can lessen their load in the moving process, tell your parents their answer should always be a resounding YES!

There are also many services ready to assist and even do the entire move for you. These companies provide a needed service for so many folks who cannot physically pack, sort, lift, sell, donate, and move by themselves. These companies work by the hour and will give an estimate for the entire move. They will even go to the new home and unpack. That is full service!

Knowing that others will help makes the task feel manageable and the decision obvious. Ask!

THE MURRAY FAMILY'S STORY

CONNIE TOOK ON the onerous task of trying to get Mom and Dad to focus on downsizing. As she states, "The painful process of sorting through and paring down possessions that meant so much began half-heartedly by Mom, more gung-ho by Dad, with items set aside for family to look at prior to having a sale or donating them.

"Shortly afterward, a unit opened up putting both parents in a panic (along with us). However, it wasn't the best location in the building for them. They really didn't want to move that quickly, so it was very hard on them to realize it probably would be sooner than the year or two that they had envisioned.

"Part of that inability to see the move coming sooner was all the accumulations that had to be gone through and sorted. At times, Mom would be in tears, and Dad would lash out (neither is a pleasant thing to experience). However, both would compose themselves in a matter of minutes, and we would tell them we loved them. This quick opening gave us the kick we needed to set goals of going through items."

Connie would go over several times a week for a few hours at a time, so as not to wear Mom out, giving her sorting assignments to be completed before the next visit. At least one of the other daughters would come weekly, and on those occasions, the length of time we worked was longer so that more would be accomplished. After about six weeks, we packed up what we had set aside for sale and headed to Rummage-A-Rama. It gave us all a goal and also allowed us to get items out of the house and garage that they were not going to keep. This was a very important step for them to take.

Meanwhile, two units at their chosen community were offered, and they agreed to the suggested move date of three months later. We all took a respite from their sorting/paring down until after the holidays and then picked up where we left off.

The sorting went faster if Mom was given a choice: which two of these five cookie sheets do you want? Which set of Christmas dishes do you use the most? As Connie states, "It's difficult to realize that many of the items you cherished so much won't go to your family as heirlooms, or the valued silverware set will only be bought for its silver value, not as a table setting. Mom did not want to choose, she wanted it all, even though many items had not been used for years or had been forgotten about. Dealing with the memories of who gave them an item, or where they were when they purchased it makes for a very emotional, slow, trying process."

As we finished going through cabinets, we would mark them "leave" or "move." It also served as a way of showing the parents how much progress had been made. While we were with Mom, the sons-in-law helped Dad sort through his remaining tools and other garage items, which was a huge help as he said he did not really know where to begin.

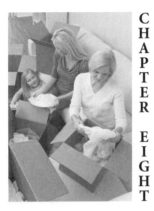

SELECTING A REALTOR

WHEN YOUR PARENTS set up a housing plan, they need to fine-tune that information about their home's value. The price they can realistically expect to get for their house will depend upon many factors, some of which they control. These include the condition of the home, whether they will improve it, when they place it on the market, and how they present the home to prospective buyers. Your parents have a choice in how and when they present their house and how much time, effort, and money they are willing to spend to get a certain price.

Advantages of a Senior Real Estate Specialist

These considerations all lead to their selecting a real estate professional with whom to work with the sale of their home.

Selling a home at any age can be an emotional and difficult task, and for you, a Realtor can handle your needs perfectly. But older adults, such as your parents, have unique issues at play and can benefit tremendously from the special skills of a Senior Real

Estate Specialist, or SRES. The designation means that Realtor has had unique training to deal with the special challenges and needs of older adults and their family. SRESs have knowledge of senior communities and the process involved in gaining admission. They have been educated in issues that especially concern those of your parents' age, such as Medicare and Medicaid, trusts, guardianships, estates, etc. They have skills in working with the many family dynamics that arise in selling what is not only the senior's home but also the whole family's home of many years. In essence, SRESs look at the bigger picture. They understand that, in addition to their role as Realtors in selling a home, they provide counsel on many peripheral issues that will naturally occur in the process for your parents. Selecting a Realtor with the SRES designation will serve you and your parents well.

Interviewing Realtors

If your parents like the Realtor they consulted previously, they may have this step covered already. If not, they should interview three agents.

What should you and your parents look for in assessing the Realtors?

- First, you want expertise and experience. What other homes have they handled in the area? How long have they been actively practicing? How familiar are they with seniors' special circumstances? Inquire about their track record. How long do houses sit with them? How does the sales price compare with the asking price? How many sales have they handled in the past year?

- Second, get references. What were others' experiences with these Realtors? Would they recommend them? Why? Get specific information that goes beyond, "She was great." What exactly did the person do that made the process a success? How did the homeowner feel during the whole sales process?

- Third, encourage your parents to listen to their inner voice. Yes, that again. What does their gut tell them? They—and possibly you—will be working closely with this person, almost intimately. Your parents must feel comfortable in this person's presence and willing to share private information as they work together through the process.

You may help here by noting how your parents interact with the different Realtors. Are they more at ease with one? Do they lean into and listen more closely to one? Do they close themselves off with crossed arms to another? Do they have a better rapport with one? What are the "bedside manners" of these Realtors?

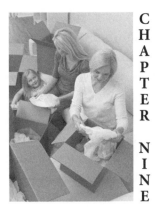

PRICING THE HOME

ONCE YOUR PARENTS have selected a Realtor, they must all work together to select a price for their home that is both competitive and realistic, based upon the current market.

Consider the Source

Your parents may think they know the right sales price for their home, but often they make the mistake of using faulty information. Every day, I meet with seniors who ask me to do a market estimate on their home to establish its value in today's market. I am often surprised at the discrepancy between the current value of my client's home and their perception of value, based on information received from sources prior to my visit.

The first misconception is that the tax bill is accurate as to the market value of our homes. Most communities are required to adjust the assessed value, usually every four years. In some communities, reassessments have not been done for a few years so those market estimates may be inaccurate compared to today's prices. Using a tax bill may be a good very general reference point, but it is not a good idea to use those values when establishing the price to sell a home or when doing estate planning.

Nor does the real estate tax bill provide reliable information for decisions about moving to a specific senior community. Relying upon the numbers in that document can lead to all sorts of problems. I have heard from many senior communities that deposits are taken, subject to the senior's home selling within a designated period of time. A large percentage of these agreements are not making it to the finish line. In the end, much time is spent on making arrangements and holding apartments, and the results are disappointing. The future resident takes the home off the market and never makes the move.

My observation is that the deal never had a chance because the homeowners used the community's assessed value as a basis for the sales price of their home. As I stated earlier, the market value on the tax bill in most cases is not accurate. In addition to not reflecting up-to-the-minute value in an ever-changing housing market, the assessment does not take into account the condition of the individual property. The assessor does not step into—or even walk around—the home in setting the value for tax purposes. Yet, much of the value depends on the home's condition. The state of a home can alter value by as much as 30 percent!

Therefore, seniors who base the affordability of a move on false information will hold to a sales price that is not realistic, guaranteeing the home will not sell. It is critical in today's market that the home start at a price that is competitive, based on condition and location. Otherwise, failure is almost guaranteed.

Another source of inaccurate information is well-meaning friends and coworkers. Yes, I suggested your parents seek out others for their opinions, but I also advised about considering the source and how that might affect the information told to them. Many senior clients with whom I meet tell me their neighbor or someone at work has convinced them of their home's value. Remember that neighbors have an emotional attachment to the neighborhood and feel they have made a good investment in their home when nearby houses sell at a relatively high price.

However, buyers do their homework (as do their sales agents), and their goal is to purchase the best home for the least amount of money. The buyers are purchasing a "house," and to your parents and their neighbors, it is a "home." Emotional attachments are normal and healthy in some respects, but they can lead to a false sense of value. Therefore, your mom and dad need to put more stock in the professionals. They will view the home objectively whereas the "expert" at work or a neighbor will too often base an opinion on emotional reasoning with no actual sales data to back it up.

Another source of faulty information can come from the media. For example, we may read a sensational headline that says sales are way up, but the fine print says prices have barely moved. Remember that the news channels seek out the sensational and, in most cases, the negative, so we get a very distorted picture of reality. The fact is homes are selling and always will in any market.

Your parents must understand, then, that the price suggested by their Realtor may differ from what they think their home is worth if they have based that value on weak information. Also, their Realtor's suggested sales price of the home will depend upon many factors. These include what homes of similar size, condition, and location have sold for recently; what homes in the area are now on the market (that is, homes that will be competing with your parents' home); and the overall economic and housing situation. Your mom and dad have little control over those considerations.

The Realtor will also address factors your parents can do something about. He or she will inspect the house more closely this time than earlier when giving only an approximate value for the home. Your Realtor will be looking for anything that might impede a sale or affect buyers' impressions of the house—structural problems, cosmetic flaws, general curb appeal, etc.—and give suggestions for improvements.

My best advice is for you and your parents to listen to the information offered by your Realtor and then voice any concerns you or they may have about the suggested price.

The Competition

Your parents may benefit from some information about their competition, the other types of homes for sale in their area, since this affects both the price they may ask and the condition in which they present their house. Expect to receive this from the Realtor; competent agents provide comparable sales and current listings to substantiate how they arrived at their suggested price.

The value of a home can vary by as much as 40–60 percent due to condition. A home in poor condition, in many cases foreclosures or bank owned, will be at the bottom of the range whereas a home in move-in condition, completely updated, will be at the top. Homes caught in the middle as to condition of the property are left in a sort of no-man's land. They cannot compete with homes in top condition as they need some updating, and they cannot compete with the pricing of bank-owned properties or short-sale properties. These homes in the middle are the ones that you see lingering on the market with "for sale" signs weathering from the changing seasons.

A home in top condition on the same block with the same square footage could sell for $200,000, and one needing updating could sell for as low as $120,000, depending on the work needed.

If your parents want top dollar, they need to listen to their Senior Real Estate Specialist (SRES) or Realtor about what steps to take to achieve a premium price.

If they want to sell as-is, that will work, too, but they must understand that the offer they receive will be far below top market value and the time the house sits for sale on the market may increase. Most sellers who choose to sell a home with work needed do not price to compete with the short sales and foreclosures and, therefore, start too high to test the waters and end up chasing the market downward. If home prices are retreating and a price starts too high, each time it is lowered, the market also is a bit lower, and that seller may never reach a price point that will attract buyers. Even if the market is going up, it may take many months to rise to their wrong price.

The best results occur when the property is offered to the public as a home in top condition or when the price is discounted for condition to meet the current market expectations. A home priced in the middle may cause the buyer to use it as a "pin ball" listing where buyers see the home and "bounce" off it to one that reflects today's buyer's expectations.

Ultimately, your parents make the choice about the asking price of their home, but remind them that they have gathered professionals for good reason—to benefit from their expert advice. These people are part of their team and are working for your parents' best interest. Certainly, their Realtor wants the highest price possible, as much as they do. For your parents to get the best results, they need to listen to their team.

As-is Cash Sale

After taking into account the work they must do and expense they must incur to get a good price for their home, your mom and dad might want an easy way out of this whole process—just sell it for cash as-is and avoid the red tape involved in selling their home in the more common way.

One popular reason for wanting to take this alternate route is that the home is in rough shape or neglected. A family member may have inherited a home that has seen the ravages of time causing damage to the structure or mechanical systems of the home. You may have heard about companies or individuals that will buy a home, pay cash, and close in a few weeks. It sounds simple and is very inviting for those who do not want to go through the process of showing the home to prospective buyers. It also circumvents typical contingencies, such as financing or, in some cases, the home inspection. But is this for everyone?

- First, if your parents are considering this type of offer, they want to make sure that the purchaser is truly paying cash for the home. We have seen many instances of purchasers offering cash, but the cash is really coming from the bank in the way of a mortgage. This will involve a lender who may put many requirements on the sale, such as repair of the home, which your parents are trying to avoid.

  Make sure such purchasers have proof of funds in their bank so you do not have to worry about the closing falling apart or a bank or mortgage company putting requirements on the sale.

- Second, as we all know, there is NO FREE LUNCH! As you may have guessed, a cash sale will be a lower purchase price. In many cases, it could be thirty to seventy cents on the dollar. That means if your parents think their home is worth $200,000, they could see offers anywhere from $60,000 to $140,000, depending on the amount of work needed. So prepare them for offers that may feel insulting. Remember, these buyers are in it for profit, as in any other business. They are looking to do the repairs, take the risk of unseen repairs, and of course, build in a profit by holding costs down.

- Third, your parents will want to have a Realtor or attorney or both view the offer and make sure that their property is being sold as-is with no warranties as to the structure of the home or its mechanicals. In other words, your parents want to make sure that once the sale is completed they are protected from future litigation. It is critical that the proper language be put in the offer for their protection.

We all want to take the easiest path to reach our goals. In real estate, as any other business, it is important to do the homework before making any major financial decisions. Your parents' Senior Real Estate Specialist can provide guidance on the pros and cons of a quick cash sale. Then they can decide intelligently as to which path to follow. For some, the home may be in great disrepair, and the thought of showing it to prospective buyers is overwhelming. The cash sale may be the solution. For others, putting the home on the market may actually be easier with the right professionals to guide them along the way. The result will depend … Your parents will need to take the time to gather all of the facts and then choose the best path.

Selling As-is versus Making Improvements

When to sell often involves a decision about whether to sell the house as-is or to sell after making improvements.

To help you and your parents make a wise choice, imagine …

A couple is considering purchasing the deluxe vehicle they have always dreamed of. Every day, they drive by car lots, and their desire for that car just grows. Finally, the time in their life arrives when they will make this most extravagant purchase. They drive to the car lot, and there it is, a gorgeous shiny new car with all of the features they have been looking for. They decide to take it for a test ride. The salesman approaches them as they inch closer to their dream ride. He greets them and prepares to open the door. But before he allows them to enter the car, he states that they should know a few important facts before the ride. "I must tell you that the engine block is cracked, but we will include a credit to have it fixed."

The couple's balloon begins to deflate.

"The wipers need replacing, and we'll take care of that. Just a little thing, but we haven't had the time. So busy, you know?"

The couple is beginning to wonder what else. If the car dealer cannot take care of such a little problem, what about bigger ones? If the dealer does not have the time for a quick job, how can he have time for more major ones?

"Oh," the salesman adds, "that dent on the passenger side? It's really nothing. Most people don't even notice it. The car's perfectly sound. And what a beauty."

Or is it? they wonder. With these problems he has told them, what others lie hidden? Apparently, the previous owner just did not care enough to maintain it.

Then, in confirmation of their worst fears, he opens the door, and they gasp as they gaze at the torn carpeting covering the floor of their shattered dream.

When purchasing anything—a car, shampoo, our dream house —we buy on emotion. We make decisions, especially one as emotional as purchasing the home we will live in for many years, based on sight, smell, and touch. A home that looks good on the outside but tired and torn on the inside will suffer in its final sales price as well as in the time on the market.

The decision to fix up or to sell as-is should be based on the reason for selling as well as the condition of the home. If your parents want to get the top dollar for their home and are willing to spend some time and money upgrading it to reflect today's décor, then spending thousands in remodeling may be the answer. However, the majority of my senior clients want to sell their homes that they have lived in for many years in its present condition.

That can work too. Just as our salesman will sell that car to someone, your parents can sell their house as-is ... to someone. Just as that vehicle will sit on the lot for some time because of its defects, so too, your parents' house will sit on the market for a while because it does not show well. And just as the price of that car will reflect its shortcomings, so too, your parents' house offered as-is will bring in a final sales price that reflects its shortcomings.

But are there improvements that should be made even when selling as-is? You bet! Have your Realtor view the home and look for structural problems, such as a bad roof, basement, siding, or concrete. Your agent can also look at the electrical, furnace, and plumbing systems to suggest a further inspection by a licensed contractor if there are signs of significant problems. Nothing will scare away a potential buyer faster than a defective basement or deteriorating roof. Realtors have the training and experience to look for possible defects and to suggest contractors with a known and reliable history. You want an honest and objective opinion so that your parents can decide whether to replace or repair a significant defect before offering the home to the public.

For example, consider a basement with a horizontal crack and possible wall movement. The standard in the industry allows one-half to three-quarters of an inch movement of the basement wall in question. More than that indicates a serious problem that should be corrected. There may also be drain-tile issues, indicated by water stains around the basement. Many times, I see mold due to drainage problems. In these cases, I would suggest a contractor or structural engineer look at the basement to determine if there is, in fact, a problem that must be taken care of. If there is not, then I make sure the owners have a report from a respected engineer or contractor to settle the fears of potential buyers. If there is a problem, then estimates can be obtained to let buyers know exactly what the problem is and what it will cost to repair.

Here is a real-life example of the inside view of a foreclosure, what will be seen as a competition to your parents' house if it goes on the market with defects intact. I warn you, it is not a pretty sight! The majority of these homes are in poor condition, both structurally and cosmetically. In most cases, it will take several thousand dollars just to start the upgrades these homes generally require.

I recently viewed one of these properties with a buyer, and what we witnessed was nothing short of sickening. The toilets and vanities were gone; the carpet was torn and emanating a pungent odor. The drywall was shredded, and the ceilings were falling. In the basement, there was standing water. And all of this was just the inside! The outside appearance was shameful. I need not go on. Needless to say, the buyer literally grabbed me and made a gesture to leave at once. This is a very typical reaction from a potential purchaser. The lesson here is that a very small percentage of buyers have the funds or even want to borrow the funds to rehabilitate such a project.

This example is extreme, but most foreclosures are variations of the condition described. Unfortunately, many of the mortgage holders of these distressed properties do not invest monies to improve the homes but, rather, let them fall into total disrepair and then sell them for less than fifty cents on the dollar. That is a real crime, and it makes no sense whatsoever. I would hope this practice of neglect would change, but there are so many fingers in the pot in these foreclosures that no one entity takes responsibility in reviving neglected homes and attracting a decent price.

Your parents do not want their home to be in such a state that it competes with foreclosures. If it does, they will suffer the same fate of losing more than half of their home's value when some updating could have brought back great returns.

Even if a home is not in the extreme situation of that foreclosed house, one with significant defects presents a great challenge in selling. To help your parents understand this, have them put themselves in the buyers' shoes. If buyers have ten homes from which to choose, they are going to consider and compare the appearance as well as the price of each. Which would your parents choose? Like any reasonable buyer, they would naturally choose the home with the least amount of repair or updates needed. Right? As buyers, your parents would want to avoid taking on the very work they now, as sellers, resist doing. So who will do it—seller or buyer?

No one really wants to do the work, but who has the most to gain from getting this done?

Buyers will walk away from homes that show a defective basement, roof, or furnace. These components of a home demand significant dollars to remedy. Usually, a home with one or more of these defects is in need of cosmetic updating also. The two combined will stop almost any sale unless the seller is willing to offer a huge discount, which in most cases is not possible.

Remember that any significant defects of your parents' home must be disclosed. If you are not selling as an estate (which may allow for an as-is sale), you must disclose any negative material information, such as a defect, that may adversely affect the value of the property. The seller cannot hide the problem or pretend he or she did not know about it. Or, if the seller does fail to disclose the problem, that failure can nullify the sale—at any time, before or after.

However, buyers are more understanding than you may think when it comes to once-in-a-lifetime events, such as a torrential rainfall in a few hours. Their home inspectors can also lessen any concerns buyers do have in such a situation and place that event within the context of what is normal and expected. Yes, buyers will still want to have the problem inspected, but they are, in most cases, fair and reasonable.

Now suppose your parents have experienced structural or mechanical problems recently and are worried about disclosing more negative news to a potential buyer. The first step in mitigating a buyer's concerns about condition is to have the problem inspected by licensed contractors. Do not get reports by a handyman or a contractor who does not specialize in the problem at hand. Get at least two estimates. If the problem is a basement issue, have them call a licensed basement contractor or inspector. This person will give them a detailed description of the problem if there is a problem and recommend a solution. If your parents have the funds to correct the defect, they should do so. Then when they sell, they are not selling a problem. Otherwise, the buyer may not be able to focus on the attributes of the home when worrying, for example, about correcting a basement issue.

If your parents do not have the funds to repair their roof, furnace, basement, or any other structural or mechanical issues, they need reliable information about the problem and how to correct it. The estimate with a written description of the problem, the solution, and the price for fixing it from the licensed contractor will at least give the buyer an understanding of the significance of the problem and give a basis for a credit to compensate the buyer.

I strongly suggest fixing the problem if it is a structural defect and if funds are available. No buyer wants to buy a problem. A defect will detract from the focus of the positive points of the home. Instead of talking about the character of the home, the sales agent will be explaining away a problem. Remember that buyers will always err on the cautious side and, therefore, estimate a doubling or tripling of the actual cost required for replacing a defect. So, if your parents have time and funds available, they will do best to fix any problems before putting the home on the market.

In summary, the final sales price your parents want will determine the path they take in preparing (or not preparing) the house.

- As-is cash sale will involve the least work, least upfront investment of resources, least preparatory time, and it will bring the lowest price.

- A house in average condition, dated cosmetically but with no structural defects, will generate a mid-range price.

- A complete remodel with updates and everything in tiptop condition will achieve the highest sale price in a relatively short time on the market.

Your mom and dad choose!

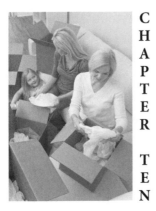

C
H
A
P
T
E
R

T
E
N

PREPARING THE HOME FOR SALE

TIMES, THEY ARE a-changing, and your parents may need a refresher on buying and selling a home. The process has changed in many ways since they bought their first or last home. The only way to advertise or get out the message about the house for sale was via hard copy in a newspaper, magazine, or flyer in the mail. Signs in front of the house were critical, as were open houses, because a buyer had no other way of seeing the interior and getting a true feeling of the listings offered.

We rarely have a face-to-face meeting with the agents we work with as offers are now delivered by email or fax. Offers are written online and emailed to the listing agent, and then we receive our answer via email or fax. Buyers and sellers can sign by clicking electronically. When we have a new listing to market to the public, it is put online within twenty-four hours to the entire world. Not only are the facts about the home on the computer, but so also is the house itself: Anyone can walk through the home via a visual tour and see the yard, exterior, and complete interior before ever calling an agent! Signs and open houses have lost their importance as savvy buyers know how to find homes online and prefer an impersonal Internet trip through the home without the pressure of an agent. A very small percentage of all sales is attributed to a sign. Using the Internet and electronic communication saves time for the seller as well as agents, with the buyer having an impression of the property inside and out before visiting the actual home.

The latest innovations are Facebook, Twitter, LinkedIn, and many other social network websites. Buyers and sellers can talk to one another in real time, as well as connect with their cell phones instantly. For real estate, this means we can reach a buyer within seconds of offering a new home on the market.

Face-to-face contact has taken a back seat to instant electronic communication and an abundance of information. The days of the handshake and smile have been replaced by a click and touch on a keypad. Advances in technology continue to bring change to all aspects of our lives. But we know one thing for certain about selling a home in today's new market. Pictures that have always spoken a thousand words now matter more than ever. Photographs of your parents' home will usually be the first view a potential buyer has of the place. The pictures of their home will speak volumes, both positive and negative. How will a buyer's online tour of their home be perceived?

In talking of what matters most in selling a home, we used to say, "location, location, location." Now we add, "condition, condition, condition."

A Realtor can guide you and your parents about what updates or repairs will attract interest to online viewers and prospective buyers touring the home in person, as well as bring the highest sales price.

One significant result of online viewing of homes for sale is a slightly lower impact of curb appeal in getting potential buyers in the door. They can see on the Internet if the interior warrants an in-person visit. So, how your parents' home looks on the inside, especially in photographs, matters more than ever.

Reasons to Improve the Home

The buyer, not the seller, determines the value of a home. What someone is willing to pay sets the market for any product, including your home.

Be aware that emotions may cloud your parents'—as well as your own—perceptions about their house. They have lived there for years, and all looks just fine to them. The place as-is has served them well for family gatherings, as well as for daily living. They probably do not see the big crack in the basement because they have lived with it for so long. It has not needed their attention, so they ignore it. The same goes for the wall paint that, over the years, has faded in spots and lost its clean, fresh look. The changes happened so gradually that your mom and dad never noticed. The decades-old kitchen cabinets do their job of opening and closing and covering the insides so your parents do not care that they are woefully out of date.

Their eyes do not see their house as a buyer would. That did not matter before, but it does now in selling their home. If your parents want success in selling at the best price possible, they will benefit by seeing it through the eyes of potential buyers—none of whom have the emotional investment. If your mom and dad's vision cannot get past the emotions and memories covering the home's defects, they will do well to listen to the advice of their Senior Real Estate Specialist, who can view the house objectively. Remind your parents that their Realtor is on their side and wants the home to bring in the highest price as much as they do. The recommendations about the home are always given with their best interests in mind. After they hear what their Realtor suggests, let them sit with the information for a while so they have time to adjust their thinking.

I have had the pleasure of helping many of my senior clients transform their properties from a tired house into an eye-pleasing home meeting current buyer's expectations. These homes have sold quickly, at a top price, and in various market conditions and won the "beauty pageant." The "price was right." These senior sellers resisted the temptation to overprice their homes because new carpet, paint, and flooring were installed. They realized that a vacant home or one cluttered with worn furnishings would not motivate a buyer so they had their homes staged with stylish furniture and accent pieces. It was one of the best investments they made. Whether you invest five hundred dollars in paint or twenty thousand dollars to stage it, the investment will always pay for itself—sometimes several times the initial investment.

If a home does not show well, it will sit on the market, waiting, waiting, waiting for a buyer, or the seller will have to reduce the price possibly several times. The first two to three weeks on the market are the most important because the listing is fresh and new for buyers to see. If they like it, they will make an offer at a price to make sure they are the lucky new owners. If the property sits on the market for an extended time, buyers will see the home as an opportunity for them to purchase at a lower price. There is no longer the sense of urgency since it has been on the market with no takers. No one wants it at that price.

The Realtor's advice may be hard for your mom and dad to hear. But they must listen to get the most from their home in the condition it is in. They cannot have it both ways. If it needs work, they will have to discount the price to attract buyers who are willing to do that work. If the price is too high, it will attract buyers who have high expectations and will simply walk out of the home (if they even bother visiting after seeing the condition that is out of line with the price in an online tour), wasting your parents' time and adding to everyone's frustration.

The condition of the home plays an especially important part when considering the likely buyers—who they are and what exactly they want. As in any sale, your parents—and especially their Realtor—must have a keen understanding of the profile of the potential purchaser of their home to make sure they present it in a way that appeals to the primary prospects.

Young people today are delaying marriage and having children later in life. This has led to the increase of single buyers purchasing on one income and a more cautious approach to their search. This group, typically twenty-five to thirty-two years of age, is looking for homes that require little updating. They do not have the funds to take on major reconstruction of the home, such as remodeling kitchens and baths or correcting structural issues. Their price range is in the lower price point of the market in the community they choose. Since this is usually their first home, they do their homework and are more educated in the real estate market than ever before, due to the proliferation of information via the Internet.

These young people often rely on their parents for financial support and for their parents' input when making a decision to buy their first home. You can imagine Mom and Dad viewing the home for the first time before an offer is made. Parents want to protect their children from making a bad choice, especially when they must make a major financial decision, such as purchasing their first home. Therefore, any repairs or upgrades needed are many times exaggerated to make sure no mistakes are made. Replacing the roof that has an estimate of $4,500 may have increased to $10,000 after overcautious parents have their say, telling their children about worst-case scenarios they know of.

Think about this. You may have children in this position. Can you hear yourself? "New roof? Oh boy. It's always more than they say. Always. You'll need new gutters, too. And downspouts. You'll have to remove all, tear it down to the rafters; you can't just put a new one over the old. You're going to be in the place for a long time; better put in the forty-year shingles. There's always damage somewhere; you're going have to replace more than you think. You always have to be prepared for the worst, believe us."

As I mentioned before, it is to a seller's advantage to repair or replace any structural defects, especially basement problems, roof, furnace, and electric and plumbing systems. Structural issues will kill a sale quicker than one can say, "Get me out of here!"

Prioritizing Work on the House

Your parents' Realtor can prioritize improvements, determining which will have the greatest impact on the sale of the home. Correcting structural defects will head that list. Next are the most important components of the home that can be considered defects if not in proper working order. These would be basement walls and drain tile, roof, furnace, plumbing, and electric. They will want to make sure all of these are in proper working condition.

If they do not have the funds to make these repairs, they can borrow the money in the form of an equity loan. A home equity loan to improve the value of their home makes good sense. Making the money work for them by upgrading the house for an eventual sale makes good sense. It will be worth the investment and save them from even more damage or repair needed down the road.

Next, look at the cosmetics. Updated, sparkling kitchens and baths bring back the biggest bang for the buck. Your parents will be amazed at the major difference they can make to the appearance of their home with a reasonable budget. I work with a company that recoats tubs at a reasonable price (much less than actual tub replacement) and can also recoat the ceramic tile. They can change that pink or turquoise into a neutral beige in one day for a fraction of the cost of total tear out and replacement. Doors of kitchen cabinets can be recovered rather than tearing out the cabinets and replacing them with new ones. Flooring in the kitchen and new carpet can totally transform your home and give it that new-home smell.

Often I hear, "Why should I replace that torn carpet when the buyer will just tear it out and put something else in its place? I'll just give them a credit." Wrong, wrong, wrong! Remember my example of the couple looking at their dream—a shiny new car with "just a few" problems. Imagine again looking at a car with torn carpet and the dealer offering a credit to replace that ugly eyesore. You know what your reaction would be, and it will be no different with a potential buyer of a house. Lighter neutral carpet with a new coat of paint on walls, ceiling, and trim can totally transform your parents' home and bring great returns, especially in a competitive market.

Painting a basement with a neutral color can change it from a dingy, depressing lower level to a bright and cheery area in which new homeowners can see themselves. It costs relatively little to have a handyman paint the basement walls and floor and will also bring back great returns. Make sure if there are any suspect cracks or seepage that your parents have them examined by a basement inspector or contractor before painting. You will not want buyers thinking you have covered up a potential problem.

By upgrading their home in a frugal and targeted way, your parents can use foreclosures to their advantage when selling. A buyer will walk through those discounted properties and then compare them to your parents' home. They will see the incredible difference between homes in distress and your parents' home, which gives a sense of a property that has been cared for. Buyers will pay a great premium for the luxury of move-in condition versus having to break the bank just to make the home habitable, let alone a home in which they take great pride.

A well-kept, well-appointed home in any market will stand out from the rest of the competition because most sellers are not willing to prepare their home just for someone else's satisfaction. Remember that homes, cars, boats, and every other commodity are bought and sold with the same principal at work ...

The buyer, not the seller, determines the value of a home. What someone is willing to pay sets the market for any product, including homes.

Staging a Home

If your parents have accepted the advice to make changes to the appearance of their home and wish to get top dollar in the market, they should consider hiring a stager. These professionals specialize in guiding homeowners to make sure their home or condominium meets buyers' expectations of colors, condition, and furniture placement. For a relatively small fee for an initial consultation, a consultant will give your mom and dad the best options to bring in the best returns. If furniture and accent pieces are needed, these professionals will stage the home with pieces they own and will charge a monthly rental fee plus their time invested in the staging process.

Stagers take a lot of the guesswork out of showing a home at its best. They know the current trends and colors and how to arrange furniture and other décor to maximize a home's good qualities. Your parents have gotten used to a couch and chairs placed one way in the living room, and it has worked well for them for many years. They probably cannot imagine any other way of arranging the furniture.

Stagers can see the possibilities and place the pieces in a new way that opens up space, gives a better flow for people moving through rooms, and helps buyers envision their own furnishings in the house.

Think about it. A three-hundred-thousand-dollar home showing average furnishings in a dated interior may sell for 30 percent less than a home fully remodeled and staged. If the stager charges 1–2 percent of the value of the home, it pays to invest in this service since the returns will be much greater than the cost of the stager. If nothing else, the consultation fee will open eyes to new and better possibilities that work with what your parents already have. Using the advice of the stager will also greatly reduce time on the market because the home will stand out over the competition.

Even if your parents do not invest in a new kitchen or bath, a staging consultant can bring those rooms to life by less costly improvements. Changing wall and ceiling colors, adding some accent pieces, and removing excess possessions all make a big difference in the home's appearance at almost no cost.

Sometimes, little changes can have a big impact in ways the owner might not realize. When viewing homes, buyers make decisions consciously using all of their senses as well as receive input from what they subconsciously take in. A clean home looks nicer than a dirty one. It also gives the impression the owners care about the house and have maintained it. Without realizing why, buyers feel at ease in such a home and subconsciously expect no surprises or hidden problems. Buyers believe the care the owners give to the cleanliness extends to the overall care of the house.

On the other hand, for example, a room too full of furnishings and knickknacks will turn them off. But they will not realize the reason—their inability to see room for their own possessions in the crowded space. Instead of using logic and saying, "All of this will be gone so I'll have plenty of space for my own things," their eyes see the clutter, and their mind tells them, "Wow! There's no room." Logic does not always prevail. Visual impact can override it. Stagers know this and work it to the home seller's advantage.

A property that shows well using calming and trendy colors and accents can evoke a sense of satisfaction, peace, and calm—and a desire to live in that home.

To find a reputable staging consultant, your parents can call their Realtor and ask for a reference of someone who has been successful in staging homes and has reasonable pricing. You will be amazed at the difference a stager will make in the whole sales process—shorter time on the market, better final sales price, smoother and easier all around, especially if your parents let the stager do much of the work. That old saying about spending money to make money holds just as true in today's ever-changing real estate market.

What to Do Now

Have you ever tried to paint the outside of a home in snow-country during the winter? Not a good idea! All too often, I visit with folks ready to make their move and put the home on the market. They are excited about the apartment or condominium they just found, and now it is time to sell their home. However, it is February here in Wisconsin, and the home needs inside and outside improvements. Downsizing of personal property has not been started, and the interior needs several upgrades before showing the home. Improvements have been avoided because moving seemed so far off … until they stumbled onto this perfect new home that they do not want to lose. The excitement has now turned into panic, and all of the seeds for high stress have been planted by their inaction to prepare their home for sale.

Avoid that scenario and encourage proactive action now.

Your parents' housing plan likely involves some work to their home. If they are ahead of the game, they can schedule repairs, painting, updating, etc. at a time convenient to them and conducive to the weather. They can even take advantage of slow periods in companies' workloads, when they may offer discounts.

For interior work, the best time is now.

One great benefit of your parents doing the improvements before they are actually ready to sell is the ability to enjoy the updates while they are still living in the home. Many of my sellers feel resentment in improving their home for someone else, someone they do not even know, and never having the opportunity to enjoy their newer, better, up-to-date home. For years, they lived with it as-is, and now that they have made it much nicer, they will move out. You can understand why they might feel upset—and why your mom and dad might prefer not to be in that situation.

Most important, your parents' preparing their home before they are ready to move offers them the freedom of moving at their leisure and without the panic of getting the home ready for sale at the same time they make a commitment to move into a senior apartment, community, or condominium. By doing work now, they lessen the chance of falling into a crisis management mode. They remain in control and have beneficial, rather than constraining, options open to them.

THE MURRAY FAMILY'S STORY

OUR PARENTS' SENIOR Real Estate Specialist informed us that to get the home ready for sale, we needed to install new carpeting, paint all interior walls, trim, etc., and do a deep cleaning from the attic down to the basement. We used a carpet installer the Realtor recommended, and a professional painter friend did the painting.

Items from the sorting/downsizing were boxed and in the garage, awaiting the downsizing/moving sale later. Connie kept some items to take to a consignment shop a few at a time. Other items were already in a consignment shop or being sold on eBay.

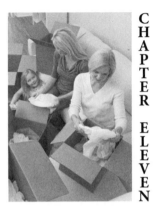

SELLING THE HOME

As you and your parents try to make sense of the current real estate situation, listen with both ears. Listen to neighbors, friends, and family when talking about purchasing their first home, selling their long-time home, or their plans to hold off or move forward. Hear all of the opinions with an open mind and an understanding of the source. Remember hidden agendas. Someone who made a poor decision in selling a home may paint a false picture in order to feel good about the mistakes made and keep others from knowing about his or her poor judgment. And remember the media's tendency to highlight the worst and ignore the good.

Most important, as I mentioned in analyzing the move, your mom and dad need to listen to their gut, their inner knowing of what is reality and what is mere gossip. So much of what we listen to is hyperbole based on either fear or lack of factual knowledge. To know the true state of the housing market, especially for your parents' part of the country, talk to the folks who live it every day, those experts I mentioned before—Realtors, mortgage lenders, senior community marketing directors—as well as those who have just sold their home or purchased a property. To have a conversation with someone directly involved and touched by the real estate market can give you valuable insight into where the market is and where it is going.

Those who do not take the advice of professionals will most often experience frustration and lack of success in selling their home. This has not changed in my more than thirty-five years of work in real estate. So, in the end, by listening to those who have knowledge based on fact and reality, a successful outcome will be the result. Those who choose to listen to people who have an opinion based on gossip and fear will pull their wings in and remain in situations that may not be healthy, mentally or physically.

Know that people will always need housing. Most people would rather live in their own home than rent. That will never change. Many reasons push people to purchase a home. These reasons will trump any market, even a down one. Our fears and our desire to move away from uncertainty too often lead to unhappy outcomes. But those who follow the advice of the experts, get the real facts, and talk to those who have recently participated in the market will be the same ones who will be later labeled lucky. Luck happens when opportunity meets preparedness. Make sure your parents are prepared and can benefit the most when opportunity comes.

Despite its up-and-down cycles, real estate has been our best financial investment over time and a great asset for retirement. If your parents purchased their home years ago, they have done quite well. A while back, interest rates were as high as 19½ percent! Can you imagine that? Not only were the rates at ridiculous levels, but also, there was almost no money available at any bank. Most lenders were shying away from the mortgage market. And yet, without a financing vehicle, we still sold homes. Yes, people wanted to buy, and people wanted to sell, so everyone got creative in figuring out how to make sales of homes work. We had a steady stream of buyers purchasing homes using alternative methods of financing. We Realtors took advantage of land contracts (a financial agreement between buyer and seller) and mortgage assumptions (mortgages that allowed a buyer to assume the terms of the seller's mortgage). The lesson is that there will always be a strong desire for young people to own their first home, as well as homeowners needing a larger home or a new home because of divorce, death, better schools, etc.

Timing the Sale

Although Realtors cannot guarantee hitting perfectly the high point of home prices, we can identify general trends that hold for most areas of the country and in most years.

Just as we are influenced in our moods and behavior by the seasons so is the real estate market. It makes sense since the real estate market is really a gathering of people who are connected to nature's changing patterns.

Can you remember when you moved? The seasons may well have played a part in the timing. Patterns of emotion that coincide with the changing seasons subconsciously guide our decisions. Our sales numbers prove this phenomenon to be quite accurate. Beginning with spring, sellers and buyers are filled with a sense of renewal. The weather changes, the flowers bloom, and people want to get outside, look at new homes, and think about changes for themselves. The spring market in Wisconsin traditionally includes the months of March to mid-June, and this holds true for most areas of the country with seasonal weather changes. As the days lengthen and warm up, we are in a better mood, life looks more promising, and we have the urge to make a change. In addition, and this is true in all areas of the country, families with children want to move before summer so they are settled in for the beginning of the school year in the fall.

We then experience a slowdown from mid-June to the beginning of the school year in September. Vacations and enjoying gardening and hobbies are at the forefront during this period.

We still do experience sales, but they are fewer as the urgency to move is lessened. Then sales pick up again as children begin their school year. This fall market typically lasts until the beginning of November.

Weather affects the sale of homes differently in each area of the country. For instance, the longer-lasting cold winters of areas, such as the Midwest, can keep buyers indoors longer than do milder temperatures of the season in the Sunbelt. Peaks and valleys in sales will occur at different stages of the seasons. An experienced agent will be able to help you use these fluctuations to your advantage.

The general trend of sales of homes in a year affects the date your parents select to put their home on the market—if they have the flexibility. They can move with the selling seasons and take advantage of the days when more purchasers are ready to pull the trigger and make a home change. More buyers always mean higher prices. We want to sell if possible when there is the greatest number of buyers available, a "seller's market," so called because sellers get to pick and choose among multiple offers for the home. The seller has the advantage. In addition to the higher prices then, your parents' closing a deal during a seller's market allows them to move during the nicer months when they can enjoy the transition as much as the buyers.

Also, if your parents are buying a new house and have the flexibility, they can wait a few months to buy during a "buyer's market," during the slower months of home sales when there are more homes for sale than there are buyers. Buyers have the upper hand because the competition among so many sellers causes home prices to stay lower than otherwise.

Your parents would want to plan their move-in date to take advantage of the seasons of the real estate market. If they intend to sell in spring, May through June would be an excellent time to have occupancy in their new home. Then they could put their home on the market in the busier months and know that they can move to their new community within the buyer's time frame. Most buyers want to close the transaction within thirty to forty-five days from the accepted offer date. If needed, their Realtor can work out an overlap occupancy where your parents can stay in their home up to sixty days after closing and pay a daily occupancy charge (usually one-thirtieth of the buyer's monthly payment). If they are timing the move for fall, they could have a move-in date of October or November and sell in the busier months of September and October.

Many homeowners looking to sell question not what month to sell but what year. With today's uncertainty, many buyers and sellers are in a quandary. None of us wants to leave money on the table. How can your parents position themselves to attract an acceptable offer when they do decide to sell?

My best advice is to begin to prepare their home for sale now. It takes a great deal of thought and preparation to market a home in the shortest possible time to attract the highest possible sale price. You know; you have seen the to-do list.

By their starting the moving process in small steps now, the end result will be a smooth, easy move to their new home. There is no substitute for intelligent planning and proper preparation!

Presenting the Home

When it comes time to offering their home for sale, your parents must have it looking as good as it possibly can at all times. Yes, many potential buyers will tour the photographs of the home online. But you can never tell when an agent will call, wanting to show the home with only a half-hour notice. Here are some tips on how to make their home most attractive, both inside and out.

- **Move first.** If financially viable, moving to their new home prior to downsizing and preparing the home for sale can make the entire sales process easier on all parties.

- **Organize the clutter.** We want potential buyers to be able to focus on the house, not on the occupants' belongings. Yes, your parents are likely still living in the home, but now they must be more meticulous than ever. Dispose of junk mail immediately, keep reading material stored in drawers, and hide away most items normally stored on the kitchen counters. Drawers and cabinets can be packed full. Closets, bookcases, and counters should give a sense of "plenty of room here." This may not be how they have lived up until now, but it should be the new protocol during the few weeks that the house is on the market.

- **Create a welcoming mood.** In the house, turn on lights in several rooms. Pleasant aromas, such as those from candles or something delicious baking in the oven, make prospective buyers feel at home. But do not overwhelm visitors with strong scents. Keep it subtle and natural. Fresh flowers always add a touch of elegance.

- **Remove furniture that is worn or no longer needed.** This was part of the downsizing that should have been taken care of before now.

- **Pay attention to curb appeal.** Have a welcoming outside, especially in front. Window boxes, flowerpots, and planters with healthy plants add beauty and style to an entrance or patio.

- **Keep windows crystal clear.** This adds brightness and conveys a sense of cleanliness.

Home Inspection

An offer to purchase your parents' home will undoubtedly be contingent upon it passing a home inspection. If they have followed the advice of their agent, the inspection should reveal few surprises.

When I started as a fledgling Realtor, we would sell a home, and the buyer would rely almost 100 percent on the seller's verbal statements as to the quality and soundness of the home. There were no condition reports. A condition report asks the seller specific questions about any problems he or she may have experienced over the years with the structural and mechanical condition of the home. Questions are direct, such as, "Have you had any water coming in the basement?" The seller fills out the form, providing information about the condition of the furnace, plumbing, roof, electrical system, and so on. If the seller has knowledge of any problems in the house or has any reports from inspectors or contractors, this information must be disclosed on the form. The buyers must sign this report, and a copy goes to potential buyers who have placed an offer on the property.

The advantage of a condition report is to lay all of the cards on the table. The buyer is made aware about any past problems and how they were resolved, as well as any potential problems, prior to beginning the negotiation for the property. In most cases, this avoids the deal falling through. Buyers are less likely to back out if they are not met with surprises.

In some cases, a condition report may not be available, such as in estates, trusts, or when the owner is not in a position to answer the questions competently (e.g., no longer lives on the property). Once an offer is accepted, the buyer typically has ten days or so (depending upon the agreement in the offer to purchase) to have the home inspected for major structural defects, such as in a basement wall, basement drainage issues, electrical violations, plumbing problems, and roof damage. If a defect is found that the buyer was not aware of, then the seller and buyer can negotiate and come to an agreement as to how to remedy the problem.

Depending on how the contract is written, whether the seller has an obligation to correct a defect or not, in the end, the buyer and seller have to negotiate a satisfactory solution—fix the problem, compensate the buyer, or end the contract. The current requirements of a condition report and buyer's inspections have worked to that end and kept the sellers and buyers, in almost all cases, out of court. When I began my career, there were numerous court cases after the closing of the sale of a home, due to either lack of knowledge of defects by the seller or failure to disclose all of the information a seller may have had, such as defects or notices received about future assessments or repairs to streets or sidewalks.

It is always best for your parents to disclose all of the information they have about the structural or mechanical integrity of their home. Since the buyer will have a home inspection, which will uncover any defects, it is better to let the buyer know about the home's weak points up front. Buyers do expect a significant number of minor issues in regards to the condition of a house. They do not want to be surprised about major issues that were known prior to the sale. Most important, the majority of transactions close with minor or no credits for repairs. If the home is priced to reflect the true condition of the home, including any problems, then reports from contractors or inspectors will satisfy the buyer.

Honesty is always the best policy, and full disclosure keeps everyone out of court. Be assured that our new laws and way of doing business are far better than the system we had prior to the requirement of condition reports and home inspections.

Moving Out

When it comes to moving, you do not want your parents to attempt this process on their own. Earlier, I suggested their getting help for the physical work in downsizing. For moving out of their home, I do more than suggest. If I could demand they let others do it, I would. The next best stance I can take is strongly advise your parents to let others take on all aspects of physically moving their possessions from their long-time home to their new living situation.

Far too many seniors make the mistake of attempting to move without utilizing the help of friends and family, as well as avoiding the hiring of services ready to assist in the move. I have seen more hospitalizations and injuries during the moving process because of stubborn attempts to stand on ladders, lift more weight than necessary, and create unmanageable stress to the point of illness or injury. Remember my story about the couple that took on all of the physical aspects of downsizing? They degenerated into two angry and physically hurting people. Now multiply that result ten times for moving everything your parents have left in their home, especially big, heavy pieces of furniture. The savings in money is not a fair tradeoff for what they will have to endure in doing this hard labor themselves. Nor is their pride in doing the work themselves worth the inevitable pain they will suffer, possibly for months afterward. As with the physical work in downsizing, when it comes to moving out of their long-time home, my best advice to your parents is:

Never say no when anyone offers to help with moving.

"I don't want to bother my children. They have enough to do." I have heard this so often and know that it is a noble intention on the older adult's part, but trying to go it alone is a recipe for disaster in too many cases. The best results for the physical move occur when a dialogue is opened (actually, is continued, if you have been following my advice about communication all along) from the parents to the children, and collaboration occurs from that open conversation. Together, the family can decide what needs to be outsourced. If your parents resist, read them that story I told in "Downsizing" about the happy couple turned ugly. They do not want that to happen to them.

The good news is that there are so many service providers that have blossomed over the last several years. I have partnered with many wonderful entrepreneurs who specialize in working with seniors. These companies offer services so needed, especially when family and friends are not able to provide the help necessary for the move. I work with sorting-and-packing companies, stagers,

movers, contractors, estate-sale companies, senior financial planners, estate attorneys, and so many other ancillary businesses that
have the senior's best interests in mind. And so does every good
Realtor. Providing connections to reliable and usually reasonably
priced businesses that will help in the move is part of the service
your parents' real estate agent offers. Going it alone is no longer
necessary or the only option when family is not available.

Here is another story to counter that one about the no-longer
happy couple.

A husband and wife, who had purchased their home from me
many years ago, remembered me and called for my help in
selling their home and moving them to a senior community.
The husband had some physical limitations, and his wife had a
medical condition that would not allow them even to consider
lifting and sorting the years of accumulated personal property
... their treasures. They wanted to take the items for their new
apartment and leave the rest for disposal, charity, or estate
sale. We had a sorting-and-packing company help them pack
dishes, books, and personal items, as well as coordinate the
mover. The couple even drew a picture of the new apartment
and guided the company as they decided what to take and
what to leave.

They successfully moved into their new apartment.

Then this same company removed items that cluttered the
interior and moved furniture so that the property showed its
best. We sold it in a few weeks and then planned an estate
sale. That was done prior to closing. After the sale, the home
was clean and ready for the new owner. The sellers received
two-thirds of the proceeds from the estate sale and were now
comfortably situated in their new senior community with no
physical issues from the move. They were pleased that they
had sought out help and were amazed at how simple the
move had been.

Which story will your parents make as their own?

The bottom line is that they do not have to do it all by themselves. With the help of family, friends, and service providers, a move from a long-time home no longer has to be overwhelming. They are never too old to learn to say, "Thank you. Yes, I would love your help."

THE MURRAY FAMILY'S STORY

WE HAD FOLLOWED our parents' Realtor's advice for preparing the home to make it look its best, including tackling the downsizing over several months. The suggested deadline of having the home ready for listing was met, and our parents accepted an offer a week later!

Previously, Mom had contracted with a senior moving company, which made a floor plan, provided packing, moving, unpacking, and setup services. It was well worth it since we knew how long it was taking us just to sort through items. We tried to have kitchen cabinet pull-outs and organizers in place before the move. Connie states, "We labeled the cabinets/drawers in the house to correspond to the labeled cabinets/drawers in the new home to make the unpacking and initial placement easier."

Our parents are settling into apartment living, starting to participate more in activities, and bring up less often the elderly family and friends who are still living at "home." Mom has even begun developing a "neighborhood" within the complex as she befriends more people, feels comfortable around them, and talks to us about their news. Mom goes to exercise class, and Dad plays sheepshead. They are going to look into Wii bowling next! Hopefully they will enjoy their sunset years even more with their new stress-free lifestyle!

Their new home requires eighteen meals per person per month, but it also has a full-size kitchen so Mom can still bake and cook, something she enjoys. It also allows them to stick to their food budget as much as possible. Another positive is that the dining requirement gets them integrated a little bit quicker as it forces them to meet new people. In addition, Susan was able to get the complex to accept a donation of Dad's pool table, which made him and the other residents very happy!

If there is one thing we cannot stress enough, it is to let your parents know how much you love them. They need to know that is the reason for wanting them to move; we want them to be safe, happy, healthy, and a blessing to us for as long as possible. Do your best to be patient and understanding, as it is a very emotional time for all family members. And always remember, as parents, they have given of themselves unconditionally; now it is time to give back, not out of obligation, but out of love. That is the circle of life.

SHIRLEY'S STORY

SHIRLEY DOES NOT mince words when she recalls the day she decided to move from her mega sized house in New Berlin, Wisconsin. Following the death of her husband, she realized the house with all of its memories and history could no longer be part of the future. The straw that broke the camel's back, however, was the four hundred dollars she paid someone to rake and remove leaves. She was vulnerable at the time and is still troubled by the transaction, she says, but does not agonize endlessly over the unfortunate experience.

The three decades Shirley and her family spent in the home were witness to the structure's gradual signs of wear and tear. It had basement problems and needed flooring, plaster, window, and door repairs and repainting. The roof had needed immediate attention a few years before and had been repaired. "I had buckets all over collecting drips," says Shirley. The condition of her house and the work required to update and maintain it convinced Shirley to find a more suitable residence.

Although she claims to being very disorganized, she tackled her dilemma with a strategic plan. Shirley made a mental note of all of the housework, repairs, and babysitting of contractors hired to do the work. "I had to be on them all of the time. You know," she confides, "they never show up when they promise. That just wasn't for me. I have too many other things I prefer doing—like sewing, bible study classes, visiting my grandchildren, and having the option of traveling to other parts of the world." She refers to a recent missionary trip she and twelve others took to Belize in Central America.

Her course of action was to downsize the home's contents and find a suitable place to live. This was, after all, a major change in her lifestyle and had to be done judiciously.

Shirley now lives in a 970-square-foot senior apartment close to the church where she attends services and close to her doctor and dentist. It has two bedrooms, two baths, living and dining rooms, kitchen, convenient laundry equipment in the apartment, and parking space for her minivan. The facility offers reasonably priced meals if desired, shopping trips, tours, and many planned activities. She has made friends and has become a helpful shopping companion to several women who are unable to get out without assistance.

Deciding to move, and the move itself, was a piece of cake for Shirley. She followed the suggestions I provided in earlier chapters for downsizing. First, she took an inventory of each room's contents. Next, family members came and took whatever they desired. After contacting a consignment center to sell any items of value, she held a rummage sale, donated to charity anything in good condition but not sold, and finally, dumped everything else. In dealing with her years of possessions, Shirley says, "Don't look back; just move. You'll never miss the stuff you didn't take with you."

This worked for Shirley, but she does confess she is not quite settled yet. She is still deciding what to do with her bell collection and her husband's camera, coin, and stamp collections.

"I'm in no hurry," she chuckles. "It's a work in progress."

Shirley took charge and made the decision to get the most out of the life she has been blessed with. Your parents, too, should assess their situation and explore those excellent alternatives that can remove today's worries about maintenance of the home, security, and health-related issues and replace them with an improved lifestyle full of more freedom. Once they do make the move, they will join the many seniors I have helped transition to new housing who declare:

"I wish I had done this sooner!"

About the Author

BRUCE NEMOVITZ HAS been a Realtor in the Milwaukee area for more than thirty-five years. When he started in the residential real estate business, there was no acknowledgement of the special needs of older adults who have lived in their homes for many years. Bruce decided to focus his business on the needs of seniors and their family when moving from their long-time home. He started a group for Realtors from all companies to discuss current topics and issues of the day and to exchange ideas and solutions to better serve the public. Since then, education has caught up with senior's special needs, and Bruce has taken advantage of the specialized certificaton. With training as a Senior Real Estate Specialist (SRES), Certified Senior Advisor (CSA), and Certified Residential Specialist (CRS), he has focused on seniors and their families for the past twenty years.

Bruce's first book, *Moving in the Right Direction: A Senior's Guide to Moving and Downsizing*, is in its second printing. It makes a handy reference for seniors while their children read Bruce's *Guiding Our Parents in the Right Direction: Practical Advice about Seniors Moving from the Home They Love*. As a contributor to *50*

Plus magazine for over ten years, Bruce has also written over 120 articles covering just about every aspect of the moving process for seniors. Bruce is a featured speaker throughout the Milwaukee-Metro area with his talks focusing on issues facing seniors and their children.

Bruce's wife of forty years, Jeanne, joins him in their senior real estate business. They have two daughters, five grandchildren, and incredible longtime loving friends.

Outside interests include playing the guitar and entertaining others through his music.

Passion permeates everything Bruce does, and he especially pours his heart into helping and guiding youth as a longtime member of the Optimist Club and as a Big Brother.